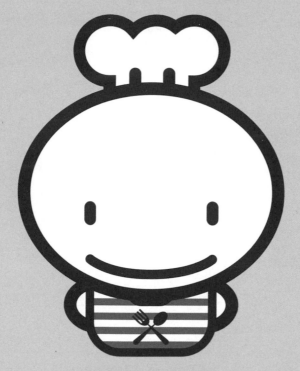

Meals Without Tears

How to get your child to eat healthily and happily

Dr Rana Conway

PEARSON
Prentice Hall
LIFE

Pearson Education Limited
Edinburgh Gate
Harlow
Essex CM20 2JE
England

ISBN 978-0-273-71268-8

Commissioning Editor: Emma Shackleton
Project Editor: Helena Caldon
Designer: Annette Peppis
Cover Design: R&D&Co
Senior Production Controller: Man Fai Lau

Printed and bound by Henry Ling, UK

The Publisher's policy is to use paper manufactured from sustainable forests.

Contents

To my husband Olly.

Acknowledgements
Special thanks to Emma Shackleton for giving me the opportunity to write this book.

Also to the people who talked to me about their experiences, read chapters and helped me along the way: my mum (Mary), my sister (Kathy), Karen Brazier, Vanessa Conway, Adrienne Cullum, Deb Futers and Karen Marshall.

Finally, to each of my three children: thanks for teaching me so much and just for being you.

What to expect from your child's eating habits

Getting your child to eat healthily amid all the temptations and time pressures of modern life can seem daunting. There are so many rules: make sure he eats five portions of fruit and vegetables a day, give him enough omega 3 foods, cut down on salt – never mind watching out for sugar, trans fats and additives. Then there are the twin dangers of childhood obesity and anorexia. How do you stop your child from getting fat, but at the same time make sure he doesn't develop an eating disorder?

Creating a healthy balance in your child's eating habits seems to be an impossible task – but it can be done. The aim of this book is to enable you to achieve this through a practical step-by-step guide to helping your little one eat well and have a healthy attitude to food, for life.

First, though, you need to think about what you should expect from your child and also from yourself. As your baby grows up to be a toddler and then a tweenie, he's bound to go through phases of fussy eating, perhaps even refusing to eat at certain times and overeating at others. Inevitably he'll also demand junk food at some stage. As for you, are you really expecting him to eat three perfectly balanced meals every day? Or are you resigned to giving him whatever he wants to eat rather than having a fight at breakfast, lunch and tea every day?

There are many aspects of your child's eating behaviour on which you can have a positive effect, but there are others that you might have to accept, however much you dislike them. Most parents should be able to get their children to enjoy a fairly healthy diet and still have stress-free meals together. You just need to follow a few simple guidelines.

The role of food and eating in our life

Food is essential for life: it provides the fuel we need to give us energy and the nutrients we require to keep our bodies functioning. So a well-balanced diet is vital for a child's growth and development, and it also reduces the risk of ill-health now, and in the future.

However, food is not just important for our physical well-being; it plays a key role in our daily routines and rituals and can also be one of life's real pleasures. When families eat together they have a great opportunity to relax and bond.

There are many things that influence which foods we choose to eat ourselves, and those which we give our children. Taste, availability and price are obvious factors, but more complex social and psychological issues also play a role. Within these, culture, religion and class are all important, as are our ideas about whether foods are healthy or appropriate for children.

Some campaigners believe that children's choices are increasingly being driven by the food industry. And this is no longer happening just through TV advertising: viral marketing techniques using websites, pop-ups, texts and emails are also

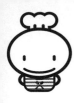

blamed for encouraging children to eat badly. In addition to these influential media, and the widespread availability of junk food, children are exposed to countless images of super-thin role models.

Given that children are faced with these powerful, yet contradictory, messages, it's not surprising that 'normal eating' is no longer the norm, and obesity and eating disorders are on the increase. Getting children to eat well is a challenge that is not to be underestimated in the face of so many negative influences, and parents need to take positive action in order to counteract them. What's more, you need to act as early as possible, since dietary habits established in infancy and early childhood will set the pattern for their diet in later life. Of course, even if you do everything right there is no guarantee you can get your child to eat healthily in the future, but by giving it a go you can greatly improve the odds.

What can you expect from your child, and when?

Few children eat exactly as their parents would like them to, and it can be difficult to distinguish real problems from normal childhood behaviours. As your child grows, her responses to meals and foods will change: messy eating, a slump in appetite and demands for crisps and sweets can all be expected at different stages. Children, being individuals, don't develop at exactly the same rate, but it can be useful, and reassuring, to know what food-related behaviour is typical for their age.

By understanding how your child's appetite and eating habits are likely to change, you should have more realistic expectations of them and therefore be better able to deal with these changes as they occur. This chapter is intended to give you a brief outline of how eating habits are likely to develop as your child grows up, and provides useful tips to help ease common difficulties. (Chapters 4 to 8 will then cover specific problems in more detail.)

Babies: weaning–12 months

Most babies take to solids fairly quickly. Initially, some might find it a shock to be offered anything other than milk and they might get frustrated that the food doesn't come in a continuous stream like milk. However, they soon learn to anticipate mealtimes and begin to enjoy the experience. At this age, babies are likely to eat pretty much anything they are offered and will have fun discovering new flavours and textures. You may find that your baby pulls a face at a certain food, such as slightly tart apple purée, but even then she will still open her mouth for more.

From about six months old, your baby will learn to grasp objects in her fist and bring them up to her mouth. She may well begin teething, too, so she might use her new ability to bite on anything she can get her hands on – and indeed on her own hands. At this age babies tend to enjoy finger foods that they can have a good chew on, such as rice cakes, but

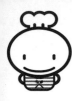

given something soft like a banana, they might simply bite off a chunk and swallow it. However, it won't be long before they learn to nibble a smaller piece and chew it, or gum it, a bit before swallowing.

Between about seven and nine months old, babies often try to spoon-feed themselves. At first very little food will make it to their mouth, but it's good to let them have a spoon (or two, if they want one for each hand) and encourage them to have a go. It will be quite some time before they can feed themselves efficiently, so you'll need to keep hold of your own spoon to help them along. Be warned that when a baby starts attempting to feed herself it will be messy, but try to resist the temptation to take over, or to wipe up too much muck until the meal is finished (see page 158).

At around the eight-to-ten-month mark babies develop, and then perfect, a pincer grip and are able to pick up small objects between their thumb and forefinger. They're often keen to practise this technique on foods like peas or bits of grated cheese, although only half of what they lift may actually make it all the way to their mouth.

Food and behaviour

A baby's appetite can easily be affected by illnesses, and even a blocked nose may put them off food for a short while. Even at this stage babies know when they're not hungry, they don't like something or they've had enough. Although you're unlikely to be faced with problems such as a refusal to eat fruit and vegetables (which is common in older children), some babies are naturally pickier than others. Also, because they are born with an innate preference for sweet foods (presumably to give them a taste for breast milk), many babies favour fruit puddings over savoury dishes.

Messy eating can be an issue, too, as your baby refines both the gross and fine motor skills involved in feeding herself. By the age of one, most babies will be reasonably good at self-feeding, but it does involve a lot of trial and error. It can get messier still when your baby begins to see mealtimes as a chance for scientific experimentation. You can't remain spotless while finding out how hard a pea can be squeezed before it pops or how warm mashed potato feels on your head!

A big problem for some parents at this stage is continued demand for night-time feeds. By about six months of age healthy babies shouldn't need to be fed during the night, but some will still wake for feeds throughout the first year, and even beyond. This demand for night feeds is simply down to the fact that they are used to getting them, and it can be a hard habit to break.

Toddlers: 1–2 years

During the second year of life, as babies turn into mobile and chatty toddlers, mealtimes will become more interactive. Your little one is unlikely to eat passively the food you spoon into his mouth as he did when he was a baby. One-year-olds can generally feed themselves – although they may still need a little help – and they often prefer to pick up food with their

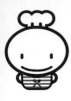

hands, be it Weetabix, rice or baked beans. So unfortunately messy eating is set to continue for some time to come.

By about 18 months, though, most can feed themselves with a spoon fairly efficiently. At first the spoon will be held in the fist like a flag and it'll be a few years before they hold it more politely, like a pen.

It's amazing to watch toddlers developing new skills, but with their increasing ability can come new feeding problems. One-year-olds often appear to eat less than they did before and seem to lose interest in food, but this is quite normal. Another common feature is more erratic eating, with a lot of food being consumed at some meals, or on certain days, and very little at others. These changes are partly explained by the slowdown in growth during the second year of life: between birth and 12 months, a baby's average weight gain is about 6kg, but during the next year it's just 2.5kg. If weight trebled in the second year, as it did in the first, your toddler would be heavier than the average eight-year-old by the age of two.

Food and behaviour

When they become toddlers, children begin to experience a growing sense of autonomy, and some will use their relationship with food as a way of expressing their independence and separateness from you. They are likely to try to take more control in many other areas of life too, such as getting dressed, washing and choosing what to watch on television. In most cases when there's a disagreement, you have the final say:

you can turn off the TV or take away a toy. However, since you can't make them eat, this is the one area where they have ultimate control.

So refusing food can become a powerful tool for toddlers struggling for independence; 'No' is often their favourite word and food battles can become common. To avoid going down this route, it is best not to make a big issue over these protests, or to force them to eat. If you do, they are very likely to fight back and demonstrate the true meaning of the 'terrible twos'. If you keep serving a varied diet with minimal fuss they may well decide to give a new, or previously liked, food another go.

It is also quite normal for toddlers to develop strong preferences for certain foods overnight, or to decide that they're no longer going to eat a whole range of foods. Neophobia (the rejection of anything new) is another common feature at this age: two-year-olds can be very insistent on having the same foods and routine all the time. This means that they need their meals served at the same time every day, and they might even demand that they always have the same cup or sit in a particular place while they eat.

Avoid the behaviour you don't want

Another feature of toddlerhood is a developing sense of humour. It can be great fun, but at times it can also be a challenge. At around 18 months old, toddlers may also find it very funny to do the opposite of what they are told. To avert bad behaviour and satisfy their appetite for learning at the same time, you can try using distractions at these moments, such as pointing out the name or colour of different foods.

Toddlers have a short attention span, and as they become more mobile they might find mealtimes restrictive and prefer to get on with more exciting activities. Some will start demanding biscuits, milk or juice, since they can eat or drink these on the go. However, this type of snacking can create problems, as it makes them too full later on to eat the nutrient-rich meals they need for their healthy growth and development. Toddlers can't understand if you tell them that a snack or a cup of milk isn't a good idea because it's nearly time for their dinner, so, again, this is when distraction is usually the best strategy.

Two-year-olds often appear negative and are easily frustrated as, despite their expanding vocabulary, they can find it hard to express themselves well. They may also find it difficult to make choices, which can be frustrating for them as they are keen to exert some power and control over what they do and what they eat. Offering your toddler limited options can help. Don't let them choose between biscuits and lunch, however, but you could ask, 'Would you like a banana or an apple?'

While many of the behaviours displayed by two-year-olds seem unreasonable, you may find little you can do to counter them. Reason, and even threats of discipline, are beyond the understanding of frustrated toddlers, and so they are likely to be more responsive to humour and distraction.

Developing minds

Around the age of two, children's speech develops rapidly and their thought processes and understanding of language become more sophisticated. As a result they often start to group together similar objects, including foods. Whereas a younger child may like carrots but not broccoli and not see any link between them, a two-year-old might. As they lump these foods into a group called 'vegetables', they may decide they dislike them all because they dislike one, or even just because they hear another child say, 'I hate vegetables.'

Increasing social awareness at this age means that toddlers take more notice, not only of what other people are saying, but also of what they are doing and eating. This means your child can be easily distracted from eating by the TV or by anyone who is around at mealtimes. Also, if a toddler sees his big brother eating a chocolate biscuit, he will no longer be content to munch on a sugar-free organic rusk. The upside of this new awareness is that if he sees you and other people eating fruit and other nutritious foods, he might well want to mimic this, too.

Pre-schoolers: 3–4 years

As children move on from the toddler years they no longer need help with feeding, except perhaps with having things like meat cut up for them. Your little one will probably eat with a spoon and a fork, although she can try to use a child's knife too, and she can drink from a cup without a lid. A bib might still

be a good idea for meals such as spaghetti, but self-feeding is now a much less messy experience. In the pre-school years children don't need to eat as often and they are able to consume more at each meal, so snacks are no longer as important as they were. Also, children are now able to understand rules – such as being allowed only one biscuit – although they may need reminding.

Once the terrible twos are over most children aren't quite as resistant to change, and they are more willing to try new foods. However, around the age of four children can be very dramatic about what they like or don't like. So you might hear them say, 'I love eggs so much, I want them every day,' or, 'I really hate peas – I can't eat them because they're too small.' This may sound fairly final, but if you don't make a fuss, then later mention how similar peas are to footballs, it might prompt a complete turnaround in opinion.

Pre-schoolers often like to mimic their parents and they enjoy helping them in small ways. So this is a good time to get children to lend a hand with the shopping and to get involved in preparing meals. By helping to wash some vegetables, or to put the topping on a pizza, they can begin to learn more about food while starting to feel some sense of responsibility too. They are also capable of learning some simple nutrition facts at this age; for example, that milk has calcium in it and calcium helps to make your bones strong.

At this age, children like to conform more, particularly with their peers or slightly older children, so they can be very influenced by someone at nursery who has visited a fast-food burger chain and has the latest 'free gift'. However, the real impact of peer pressure doesn't usually become apparent until they are in school full-time.

It is now that children need to be allowed some controlled freedom, so it's good to give them choices more often. Generally these should be between similar healthy foods, or if you're choosing biscuits in the supermarket, they might like a say in which packet to buy. However, pre-schoolers aren't yet ready to handle more complicated choices, such as whether to eat a biscuit straight away or to save it until later when other people will be having one. They're likely to want it straight away, then become very upset when biscuit time arrives and you remind them about the decision they made earlier.

The kinds of problems to expect now are those that can occur at any age – including a dislike of vegetables. In addition children may get very involved in certain activities which will make them reluctant to come to the table for a meal. Problems relating to comfort eating or overeating (though more apparent in older children) can start to emerge in pre-schoolers, so it's important for parents to continue to encourage a healthy attitude to food.

Primary school children: 5–10 years

Once children reach school age, growth becomes slower and their appetite is likely to fluctuate with activity level. This means that you might find your child eats very little for lunch if

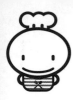

he's just been playing in the house and watching TV, but after a day out he'll come home and eat adult-sized portions.

From about six (but sometimes younger), a child's milk teeth start to fall out and are replaced with permanent teeth. Some children don't mind having a wobbly tooth or a gap, but others can become very choosy about what they eat for a while. You can understand them wanting to avoid apples if they are missing teeth at the front, but watch out for those who use it as an excuse to skip other, less favoured, foods.

Food and education

As children move through primary school and become more capable of logical, organized thought, they are better able to understand nutrition. So this is when they can learn about food groups, such as carbohydrates (for instance, bread, rice, pasta), rather than just classifying foods by colour or shape.

Children will most likely be taught some basic nutrition in school, but if parents really want them to understand healthy eating it must be made to be a part of everyday life. Learning about food, as with other subjects, is easier if it is an active process, rather than simply a lecture. Children will probably ask more questions as their desire for facts increases and they will need more sophisticated explanations about why they should eat different foods. If you know the basics yourself, you can find out the details they want together.

At this age children are increasingly eager to take on some responsibility and be useful. One way of satisfying this desire is to give them chores to do around the house, including food preparation. Becoming more involved in meals through activities like planning, shopping and helping to cook food will not only help your child to learn about nutrition and pick up valuable skills for later life, but will also give him a sense that he is contributing to the family.

These years of mid-childhood are a time to bridge the gap between previous dependence and approaching independence. Up to this point, children will have generally looked up to their parents as the source of information on most subjects, but now they are developing growing connections with other people, such as teachers and friends. They are also likely to be hearing different messages about food as they eat outside the home more often. Seeing other people's packed lunches may be quite a revelation, as your child learns that some of his friends are allowed jam sandwiches with white bread, and get crisps and chocolate biscuits every day (lucky things!).

Children might also be served different foods when they go out to tea, but this shouldn't be viewed as a problem; it's all part of the learning process which they should enjoy. So while it is important to practise healthy eating at home as much as possible, children should be able to have junk food sometimes, if they ask for it. It can actually help them to adopt a healthier attitude to eating if they are given permission to break the rules occasionally, rather than your enforcing a blanket ban.

As children become better at verbal reasoning, they are more able to think through the consequences of their actions.

For example, they can understand that if they don't eat their dinner they might feel hungry later, or that if they eat their whole week's allowance of sweets on Monday, they might regret it on Tuesday. They are also able to reason in a more sophisticated way and work backwards, perhaps realizing that a tummy ache may have been caused by over-eating.

Children often become less active as they get older, spending more time watching television, for instance. They may eat a less healthy diet, too, which can result in weight problems. Girls in particular can become increasingly aware of body image and weight control and and both boys and girls are more likely to dwell on problems with school friends, feel stressed about schoolwork and have mood swings or feelings they don't know how to deal with. All of these factors can bring about comfort eating in some children.

Establishing good habits

While many eating habits become well established in early childhood, it's never too late to tackle food problems. Research with five- to seven-year-old children has found they are surprisingly malleable when it comes to dietary improvement; and trials which used a healthy eating programme involving the 'Food Dudes' (see page 224 for more information on the Food Dudes) found that even children who expressed a strong dislike for fruit and vegetables could be persuaded to increase consumption of these foods, given the right motivation.

From about seven years of age children become capable of concrete problem solving. So if they have an issue with food, such as being overweight, they are able to talk it through and try to work out a solution with you (see page 217).

Don't forget

O Food is there to meet biological needs, but it also plays a psychological and social role in life.

O Parents can help balance the negative influences on their child's eating habits by promoting a healthy attitude to food.

O As children develop, their behaviour in relation to food and eating is likely to change.

O Babies generally enjoy a varied diet and gradually begin the messy process of self-feeding.

O Fussy eating and a slump in appetite often occur in the toddler years, as growth slows down and children try to demonstrate their increasing independence.

O Pre-schoolers are independent eaters and need a limited amount of choice about what they eat.

O During the school years, poor eating habits and a lack of physical activity can become problems. However, children at this age are increasingly responsible, better able to understand nutrition and can get involved in solving any problems they might have.

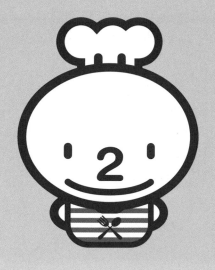

What is stress-free parenting?

Bringing up children can be incredibly rewarding; but it can also be very stressful when situations get out of control. Mealtimes are no exception, and they can be exhausting if your little one won't do what you want her to.

Perhaps your daughter refuses to eat her vegetables, try anything other than chips, or stay at the table long enough to consume more than a couple of spoonfuls. Maybe she gobbles down everything on her plate without pausing for breath and immediately demands more, or perhaps your toddler hurls your lovingly prepared food all over the floor. Whatever the problem, it can be frustrating for you and it can make mealtimes stressful for everyone. However, it doesn't have to be that way: the key to enjoying harmonious mealtimes is in how you respond to your child's behaviour.

Let it go

When you are trying to get your child to eat vegetables you might start by using the power of suggestion: for example by saying, 'These carrots taste lovely.' Then, if this doesn't work, you might move on to gentle persuasion such as, 'Why don't you try them? – you might like them.' Next, you'll probably attempt logic: 'Eat up, they're good for you.' As your anxiety levels increase and you wonder whether your child will ever consume even a single portion of the recommended 'five-a-day', you inevitably resort to bribery: 'If you eat your carrots, you can have ice-cream for pudding.' Finally, realizing that none of these approaches is working, you pop a few slices into your child's mouth, then try to hold back your anger as he promptly spits them out.

There is an underlying problem with all these methods though: it is impossible to manage the eating process this way, and if you do try, it will just lead to stress. If you have attempted any or all of the above, don't worry – you are not alone. But you might get better results if you take a different approach.

When you are away from a mealtime setting you could try to teach your children about good food and basic nutrition. Also you could try to eat together as a family, at a table, regularly, and without distractions such as the television. Keep serving them healthy meals, but when you put their plates down, you have to let go and accept that you can't control what they put in their mouth.

If you give your children responsibility for what they actually eat, and focus instead on maintaining a pleasant mealtime environment, the stress should melt away. Or at least it should decrease enough to allow you to bite your tongue instead of saying, 'Be good and finish it up' or 'Just one more spoonful.'

If you follow the five dos and don'ts over the next few pages you might be surprised to find that mealtimes can actually be quite enjoyable experiences. As you begin to relax, so will your children, and if they do, they'll be much more likely to eat well.

1 Lead by example

Children tend to eat what they see other people eating. The food culture they grow up in has a major impact on their diet – just think about Australian Aborigines munching on insects or South American Indians eating monkey.

Our environment even determines which combinations of foods are acceptable. For example, your child probably eats meat and chocolate but never at the same time, although this is the basis of a popular recipe in Mexico. The time of day at which we eat certain foods also varies culturally: while most British children wouldn't want boiled rice first thing in the morning, it is a staple breakfast for many youngsters around the world.

Your children's feelings about food come partly from what they see in the shops, on television or in other people's homes, but undoubtedly the biggest influence comes from what they see you eating and what is available in your household.

There is little point in telling them to eat well if they don't see you doing it. Research has found that when mothers put pressure on their daughters to include more fruit and vegetables in their diet without leading by example, it doesn't work and they will actually eat less. However, when daughters see their mothers eat more fruit and vegetables themselves, so do they.

This clearly demonstrates that what you do is more important than what you say.

2 Offer a healthy balance of foods

It seems obvious, but if you don't give children healthy meals, there's no chance of them eating healthily. If you serve chicken nuggets and spaghetti hoops every day, for example, you can't blame youngsters for not eating fruit and vegetables.

You also have to make healthy eating the rule rather than the exception. Children are unlikely to go for vegetables when you suddenly serve them up one day just because you've made a New Year's resolution, or you've heard a scare story about childhood obesity. They need to be given a healthy balance of foods, including vegetables, every day if they are going to accept this as the norm.

Remember, you're not punishing your child; you're doing him a favour and setting him up to eat well in later life. A good diet now will provide a lifetime of health benefits. Of course, he probably won't thank you for your concern, but if you let him eat over-processed foods containing lots of fat, sugar and salt, he may well blame you later if he turns into an overweight couch potato!

It may seem a waste to peel, chop and cook carrots your child may not eat, but if you don't you're not giving him a chance to learn to like them. If you are eating together (see page 31), it is very little trouble to prepare a few extra slices and put them on your child's plate, or you could just cook him a very small portion.

Snacks, as well as meals, should be healthy. Biscuits, cakes and crisps are fine for an occasional treat. But since snacks

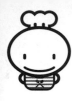

make up such a significant part of our children's diet, particularly for the younger ones, those that they have every day should be nutritious.

So encourage healthy eating among all members of your family, but try not to make a big fuss about it. Being over-enthusiastic about a particular food might actually turn your child off it, whereas if you just treat it as a normal part of life, he is more likely to accept it.

3 Teach your child about food and nutrition

In addition to being given nutritious food, children need to learn about what different foods do for their body; and they can begin to understand simple nutritional messages as soon as they can talk. Only when they have this information will they be able to make good food choices and take some responsibility for keeping themselves healthy. You might need to read up on the basics of nutrition yourself before you start, but it's worth the effort. If your child thinks a doughnut filled with strawberry jam counts as a portion of fruit, she has little hope of choosing a good diet for herself.

While you need actively to promote nutritious foods to counteract messages about the delights of junk food, it's also essential to maintain a balanced attitude. You don't want healthy eating to become an unhealthy obsession, or for your child to become fixated on illicit snacks. It is perfectly possible to explain the benefits of fruit, vegetables and milk without demonising chips or chocolate. In the same vein, it's better not to talk in terms of 'good' and 'bad' foods; all foods can be included in a healthy diet, but you need to impress upon your child that she should eat much more of certain foods than others.

(Chapter 9 provides ideas for getting your child involved in planning meals, shopping for food and helping to cook it. These activities will help children develop the skills they will need if they're going to eat well in later life.)

4 Eat together

If you've tried to sit down for the occasional Sunday lunch with your children, it might have put you off the idea of family meals completely. But think about the experience honestly – could this have been due to your unrealistic expectations? Parents who don't usually eat with their children sometimes have an idealized image of the occasion: they serve up a delicious three-course meal which they assume will be gratefully enjoyed by all. However, if the food doesn't come at the children's usual mealtime, includes things they're not used to, or means they have to stay at the table for more than their usual five minutes, it's unlikely to be a great success. The occasion, which may have started out as a novelty for them, could even end up with tantrums and indigestion all round.

However, if you try to eat together more regularly you will find out what works well for your family, and these meals should become a far more enjoyable experience. If you have

The benefits of family meals

O Children have a better diet. Research suggests that youngsters who eat with the rest of their family consume more fruit and vegetables, grains, fibre and vitamins and minerals. They also have less fried food and saturated fat. This is probably because children's tea often involves 'kid's foods', such as fish fingers or burgers and chips, which are easy to prepare and guaranteed to be eaten. Any 'proper cooking' tends to wait until after the children have gone to bed, because most parents don't want to cook two evening meals from scratch, and so it tends to be the children who miss out.

O You can be a role model for healthy eating. Children are more likely to eat and enjoy nutritious food if they regularly see you doing the same. In particular, those children who won't try new foods are usually more willing to do so if they see someone else taste them first.

very small children, mealtimes probably won't be leisurely and relaxing for a while yet, but it's still a great opportunity to enjoy good food and each other's company and to teach children to do the same. Eating together as a family, even if it's just a family of two, should be a special time that you look forward to, not dread. Unfortunately, less than a third of families share a meal more than once a week, which is a shame, because it can be a hugely rewarding experience.

O Eating together develops communication skills – children learn how to listen to others and share their opinions and ideas. Research from Harvard University has shown you can have a greater impact on your children's language development by having family dinners than by reading with them.

O Eating together promotes good manners and helpfulness. If children see you eating with a knife and fork, and not talking with a mouthful of food, they are more likely to do likewise. It will also benefit those who find it hard to sit still long enough to eat a proper meal.

O Shared mealtimes help you to bond as a family. It may be the only time of the day when all of you are in the same room, let alone having a conversation together. Any meal eaten this way, no matter when it features in the day, is a good time to talk about what you've all been doing and to make plans together.

If you get into the habit of eating with your children now, the benefits of doing so will last well into their teenage years. In fact, research suggests that those teenagers who frequently eat with their family are less likely to smoke, drink or use marijuana. They also perform better in school and are less likely to become depressed.

For many families, working hours and after-school activities make it impossible for them to eat together every evening.

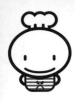

In addition, a quarter of British families don't have a table they can sit around. Nonetheless, you should be able to share at least some of the 21 meals children have a week, even if it is just breakfasts or weekend meals. If space is the problem, why not use a folding table? Then, even if you can't actually eat with your children, you can at least sit with them for a drink or snack and a chat.

5 Relax and trust your child

This may be easier said than done, but it will help if you hand over eating control to your child, along with his plate. Reassure yourself that you are doing as much as you can to help improve his diet in other ways, and if you do start to feel yourself getting stressed or wound up, stop and think, 'Does it really matter?' Even if your child eats nothing at all for one meal, he's not going to starve; he may be hungry later, but that will help him learn to eat when food is on offer.

Nagging and hovering are not going to encourage a child to enjoy meals, and since they're not effective, these techniques will serve only to increase your stress levels further.

As children get older they need to become more involved in making decisions about what's for dinner or what goes into their packed lunch. The options should be limited at first: for example, ask your child, 'Which of these two vegetables do you think we should have tonight?' Once children get older, though, they need to be given more opportunities to make choices for themselves.

Don't

1 Make a child eat anything

You should never force a child to eat anything, whether physically or with bribery, threats or guilt trips. This can be tempting to do, because when a child eats well it's often seen as a sign that she's healthy and thriving and that you're doing a good job as a parent. However, your responsibility is to provide her with good food, not to make her eat it. When a child tells you she's had enough, you need to respect the fact that she knows better than you how she feels. You can insist a child stays at the table while other people eat, but you shouldn't force her to eat anything if she doesn't want to.

Very young children are good at knowing when they've had enough. By insisting a child eats more, you are telling her to ignore her internal body cues, which is what usually happens as children grow older. Research has shown that between the ages of three and eight, children become less likely to stop eating when they feel full, and more likely to overeat when offered a food they enjoy.

You can help your child to stay in touch with her body and its needs by encouraging her to recognize and respect when she is hungry or full, and by listening to what she tells you. Insisting on 'just one more spoonful' is going to make no difference nutritionally – it won't ward off scurvy or make a child grow taller. It might make you feel better, but it still gives a child the message that she should eat when she doesn't want to. By showing your child that you trust her, she will

learn to trust herself more. It doesn't mean you should never encourage your child to eat, but be wary of forcing her.

2 Label your child

Try to avoid referring to your child as a 'picky eater' or a 'crisp monster', either to his face or to other people, when he is in earshot. Using a negative label or describing a child as hating vegetables or having a sweet tooth can make any eating problems worse.

It's easy to make these kind of comments without thinking, but you don't know what will stick in his mind. If a child hears that he hates fruit and won't even taste it, he's very likely to believe it and then the idea will become firmly established in his head. Instead, try focusing on his positive behaviours and give him praise for anything he does well; for example, don't comment on the uneaten peas on his plate, but praise him for eating the carrots.

When you label a child in your own mind, it can also affect the way that you feed him. For example, a child's dislike of fruit may just be a passing phase and partly due to his age. Perhaps he is bored with the apples and bananas he's always offered, but he might love peaches, grapes or some other fruit. By labelling him you are subconciously making it unlikely that you will keep offering the usual fruit (that he may well return to later on), or provide the opportunity for him to try new ones. On the other hand, if you maintain an open mind he'll be more likely to do the same.

3 Be too rigid with your child or yourself

No food should be banned – unless your child has an allergy or intolerance to it. Food should be an enjoyable part of a child's life and no one should feel guilty about the odd treat or what they eat at parties and other special occasions.

Limiting access to high-fat and high-sugar foods seems an obvious way to get children to eat a healthy balanced diet. However, research has shown that forbidding certain foods can draw a child's attention to them and also make them appear more attractive and desirable.

Likewise, trying to limit a child's overall food intake can backfire on you. You might do this because she is overweight or you have a weight problem yourself and want to help your little one avoid the same fate. However, it can result in your child becoming preoccupied with food, and so overeating when she gets the chance out of fear that this is her only opportunity to eat.

Parents, especially mothers, can set strict rules about what they let themselves eat – but go easy on yourself. If you try to limit your own food intake and never eat foods that you really enjoy, your child will witness this. She'll also be able to see when you inevitably eat the chips or chocolate you were denying yourself.

Eating treats shouldn't be linked with failure; they are absolutely fine as part of a healthy diet. A balanced intake doesn't have to work on a meal-by-meal basis, and for some children

it doesn't even work on a day-by-day basis, but over several days – since they might favour particular foods over others on certain days.

So when considering your child's diet and what it should include, set realistic standards. Aiming for unachievable goals will only lead to stress and guilt.

4 Give children food as a reward or for comfort

Many parents offer their children sweets or other high-sugar or high-fat foods as a reward for good behaviour. These treats can seem to be the ideal incentive for 'good' behaviour – whether it's learning spellings, tidying up the bedroom or not hitting each other in the shops. Sweets are easy to buy, cheap and they're usually very effective at bringing about immediate short-term changes in behaviour.

Unfortunately, the disadvantages of using food as a reward far outweigh the short-term benefits. If you give your child chocolate, sweets, crisps and cakes, he will eat less of the foods which provide iron, vitamin C and the other nutrients needed for healthy growth and development. Research has also shown that when a food is presented as a reward, a child's liking for it increases significantly and it also encourages over-consumption of these foods, which can contribute to weight gain.

In addition, giving sweets as a reward for good behaviour can have long-lasting ill effects. By offering them in this way, it undermines anything you say about how great it is to eat a well-balanced diet. If healthy eating helps children to feel fit and well and to run, jump and concentrate, then why give them unhealthy foods when they're good? Eating sweets as a reward can also stop children from learning to respond to their own hunger and satiety cues and in turn encourage them to eat to reward themselves, even if they're not feeling hungry.

Alternatives to food rewards

- Playing a favourite game with parents.
- An extra book at bedtime.
- Stickers.
- A magazine.
- A balloon or a pot of bubbles.
- Hairgrips, finger puppets, plastic animals, and so on. Buy a set and give them out one at a time.
- Drawing or art materials, such as glitter, felt pens, paint.
- A video or DVD. You can borrow them from libraries or buy them cheaply from charity shops.
- 'Points' towards a bigger reward: for example, your child collects 10 stars on a chart and gets, say, a swimming trip, new football or a book.
- A 'certificate' to display on the wall.
- Help phoning Granny, or someone else. The child could then tell the person about their achievement.

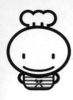

Children don't need to be given a reward every time they achieve something or behave well; praise and thanks from a parent are often as highly valued by a child. Or when an incentive is needed to make your child do something you could promise to spend extra time on an activity your child enjoys, or offer him some other form of non-food reward.

Likewise, using food to comfort children who are hurt or upset gives them the wrong message about when and why they should eat. It can promote emotional eating and encourage them to consume food when they're not hungry but want comforting or to feel good, which is associated with unhealthy eating habits and weight problems in adulthood. Comfort eating can start at a very early age and can become worse as a child gets older. Children can enjoy, say, birthday cake and Easter eggs without any risk to health, but if they turn to such foods regularly to cheer themselves up, it will cause problems.

5 Allow too much TV

Watching too much television is thought to be detrimental to a child's health for several reasons. A number of studies from around the world have linked TV viewing to weight problems. A study in the Bristol area found that three-year-olds who watched more than eight hours a week were more likely to be overweight at the age of seven. Another study in New Zealand, which followed children from five years old, found that the more time they spent watching TV in childhood, the greater the chances they had of being overweight and unhealthy in adulthood.

There are several reasons for this link: part of the problem is that kids often eat unhealthy snacks while they watch television and they also see adverts for junk foods, which they then want to eat. In addition, the more time children spend watching television, or on the computer or games console, the less they have for physical activity. In fact it has been found that children who spend more than two hours a day in front of a screen are most at risk of being overweight. Therefore, experts believe that two hours per day should be the absolute maximum for children – and that includes time spent on the computer or games console, as well as watching television.

Relieving the stress

If your child has a particular eating problem, such as spitting out food or refusing milk or vegetables, it can be hard not to get stressed and to dread meal times. Chapters 4 to 8 address specific problems and give tailored solutions. However, the issues raised in this chapter will come up again and again, as they are the key to developing good eating habits. By focusing on these and trying to change any bad habits you may have, such as nagging at mealtimes, you should be able to see positive changes in your child's behaviour around food.

This process can be hard and you will sometimes get it wrong – because all parents do – but keep going back to the dos and don'ts listed here and you should be able to get back on track and begin to make progress again.

Don't forget

O Stress results from trying to manage exactly what your child eats, but being unable to. You can't control what she actually puts into her mouth, so if you accept this, your stress levels should reduce.

O You can encourage healthy eating by teaching children about food and nutrition and providing healthy meals in a pleasant environment.

O You can help your child to form a healthy relationship with food by recognising when he is hungry or full and by not using food as a reward or for comfort.

O If you set realistic standards for what you and your child eat, mealtimes should become more enjoyable and less stressful.

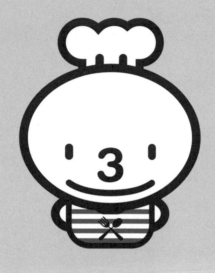

How do you feel about food and eating?

Our own relationship with food has a big impact on how we feed our children, and our attitudes to eating are complex. Some people have food on their mind almost all the time – even while they are eating a meal they are planning the next; or they finish and feel guilty about having too much and vow to 'be good' in future. Others rarely think about it: only when their stomachs start growling does it occur to them that they might like to eat.

A person's relationship with food starts at a very early age: you may recall experiences in your own childhood that led you to hold certain views on eating. Many people believe that wasting food is tantamount to a criminal offence, and so they think they must finish everything on their plate, no matter how full they are. You might have been encouraged to think this way through tales of less fortunate children, or being made to sit at the table until your plate was empty. If so you probably want your own child to clean her plate too. You might not use your mother's line about the starving children in Africa, but if you cajole your child to have 'one more spoonful', and then 'just a bit more', you are giving her the same message: that good boys and girls should eat up everything no matter what.

It's worth looking at your own relationship with food and considering how it affects the way you feed your children: not to make you feel guilty, but to help you see how you can change your attitude and maybe improve the situation. Of course, fully understanding these issues could take years of psychoanalysis. Nobody's relationship with food is simple: it can be a friend they turn to for comfort, or an enemy that needs to be kept in check, or even both. Issues surrounding feeding and mothering just add to this complexity.

What role did food play in your childhood?

Becoming more aware of the positive and negative associations you have with eating can help you to separate your own issues from those of your child; and by doing this you may come to realize that what you perceived to be a problem, such as not finishing meals, is not really worth worrying about.

To understand your feelings about food you should first look at the role it played in your upbringing. So take a few minutes to think about the five questions below:

O What were mealtimes like when you were a child?

O Were your parents concerned about their weight?

O Do you remember any negative comments or bullying about your size?

O What happened when you didn't finish a meal?

O How do you think your mum felt about feeding you?

Now consider how you feel about these experiences and how they might have affected you and the way you eat now.

Your mother may have felt that cooking and feeding the family was a labour of love. If she enjoyed preparing your favourite meals and seeing you eat them, it might have made you feel valued. But it could also have led you to equate food with love and turn to it for comfort. Alternatively, you might have felt guilty if you didn't finish her lovingly prepared meals.

Perhaps your mother saw it as her job to police your food intake, so she banned sweets and force-fed you vegetables. She may have worried about you not eating your greens and so insisted that you sit at the table until you finished every last bit of cabbage. If this was the case, did it teach you a lesson? Do you now eat greens with every meal? The answer is most likely 'no'.

As you think about the way you were brought up and fed, you will probably begin to see a connection between it and your current relationship with food. Of course, you might have been fortunate enough to have had a mother who had a fairly balanced, healthy and flexible approach to food, which you have also adopted. Alternatively you might have disliked her approach and so decided to do the exact opposite with your own children.

Our attitude to food isn't just the result of our upbringing. It is also affected by our later experiences: for example, how friends, flat-mates or others around us ate, what we've read or seen on TV and how we think other people see us. So consider these questions, too:

- Have you ever eaten just because you felt stressed, lonely or upset?
- Do you eat whatever you like?
- How important is healthy eating to you?

- Have you ever had an eating disorder?
- How do you feel about your weight?
- How much time do you spend thinking about what you've eaten or what you might eat?
- How do you feel about your child's size and diet?

Taking a closer look at the role that food has played in your life may help to explain why you now hold certain beliefs, and it should also help you to appreciate the lasting impact you will in turn have on your child's eating habits. If your current relationship with food is not as healthy as you might wish, now is the time to think about whether you are passing on similar feelings to your child, and to re-evaluate your attitude and approach. Also, consider whether the way you currently feed your children is really going to make them eat well in the future.

So how do your weight and eating habits affect those of your children?

Several studies have looked at the way parents, particularly mothers, influence their children's eating habits. Clinical problems are often passed down through generations. A woman with an eating disorder is more likely to have a daughter with an eating disorder, for example, and a child with an obese parent is at least three times more likely to be obese when he grows up.

Critical issues of control

When it comes to obesity, genetics undoubtedly play a role, but there are other important factors too. Children whose parents are overweight or obese may have a less healthy diet and a less active lifestyle than others. However, it is not simply a case of parents passing on their unhealthy habits. A study of mothers and their five-year-old daughters found that women with weight concerns were more likely to try to restrict their child's intake of high-calorie foods – presumably in an attempt to stop their daughters developing the problems that they themselves had. However, what actually happened was that these girls appeared to become less able to regulate their own food intake, so the strategy backfired.

In the study, girls were given a high-calorie drink before lunch to see if it led them to reduce the amount they ate. While most girls compensated by eating less lunch than usual, those with more restrictive mothers were less likely to reduce their intake. Their bodies should have been telling them that they didn't need to eat so much, because they were fuller, but the girls weren't receiving or weren't responding to the message. In another experiment the same girls were given a range of snack foods, such as crisps and biscuits, when they weren't hungry. Once more, those with larger and more restrictive mothers were found to eat more, again demonstrating a lack of self-regulation. It seemed that the mothers' strict control actually made their daughters more likely to overeat when they got the opportunity. Perhaps they hadn't learnt to tune into their own hunger and satiety signals, and hadn't had the chance to learn how to make sensible choices about food.

While the five-year-old girls in the study probably didn't get many opportunities to overeat, older children often do. When they start to have meals away from their parents and get greater access to food, weight problems can begin or worsen if they exist already. Studies have found that children who aren't allowed sweets, crisps or similar foods can become obsessed with them. This type of ban can result in secret eating or hoarding. Eventually these children may be unable to control their eating, which can lead to bingeing and yo-yo dieting.

Loosen the dietary reins

All children should be allowed treats occasionally, and they will inevitably overeat at times. Though it can be difficult, parents sometimes need to take a step back and allow their little ones the space to make choices and mistakes. By allowing children a greater degree of control over their own diet, feeding problems such as overeating can often be reduced.

Research into how mothers with eating disorders feed their children has found that issues of control are critical. In one study in Oxford, mothers with eating disorders were found to be pushier when feeding their one-year-old babies and there was more conflict.

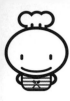

Another study looked at women and their four-and-a-half-year-old children in the Reading area; it showed that children of mothers with disturbed eating habits (though not necessarily with a diagnosed eating disorder) were more likely to have feeding problems.

When the researchers tried to find out how these eating problems were passed on they came up with some interesting findings. Mothers who were over-concerned with their weight or who displayed characteristics of eating disorders didn't give their children such organized meals; they were less likely to be fed at regular times or at a table, and they were more likely to have the TV on while eating. These mothers also tended to be controlling in their relationships with their

Parental pressure

Although most research has focused on mothers, the impact that fathers have on the way their children eat shouldn't be ignored. A girl's father is often the most important man in her life in childhood and negative comments about her weight or appearance can have devastating effects on self-esteem. A study of children of normal weight found that those who believed their parents wanted them to be thinner were three times more likely to think they were fat. There is evidence that criticism about weight, shape and eating in childhood can have long-lasting negative effects.

children, and there was more conflict at mealtimes and in other activities.

This would suggest that children can benefit from structured meals at the table, combined with a more relaxed maternal attitude to what they actually eat. In this way, they will be more likely to develop a healthy relationship with food.

The way forward – food and your child

Thinking about your relationship with food may have brought up issues you hadn't considered and perhaps don't know how to deal with. But hopefully this self-exploration will help you to see how your actions can have a negative or a positive impact on your children and the way they see food. (If you feel that you need help to avoid passing on problems to your child, such as an eating disorder, see the resources section at the back of the book for useful contacts.)

You may never be able to resolve your own food issues, but you don't have to in order to give your child a more positive approach to eating. Simply acknowledging your own relationship with food can help you see any mistakes you might be making. For example, if your child is an erratic eater – eating well some days and having very little on others – you might feel anxious that his eating is out of control and try to regulate it. However, by looking at yourself you may realize the anxiety you feel is a result of concerns you have about controlling

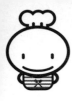

your own eating. In that way you can allow yourself to step back and see that if your child's eating habits are not really a problem for him nutritionally, why worry?

Choosing the best approach

You might be starting to think the best strategy is to let your child eat whatever he likes, or you may have already decided not to try to control your child's eating because your mother was strict about food and you vowed to do things differently.

It might seem the easiest option in some ways, but leaving complete control to your child is not the answer. It's not healthy for a child to have burgers and chips every evening, which is what they may well choose given free rein. Kids *need* structure and they also need to be given only a limited amount of choice, which, if they are to eat healthily, must come from a predominantly healthy range of foods.

If you picture yourself lovingly preparing nutritious meals that your children enjoy and thank you for, think again. Perfection rarely happens, so it's better to set realistic standards for your child's eating and for your own. We can be incredibly hard on ourselves and set unattainable, or at least unsustainable, dietary standards – such as vowing never to give in to a weakness for crisps or biscuits. By being easier on yourself and flexible about what you let yourself eat, you will be able to relax more about your child's eating. Also, remember that whether or not your child enjoys broccoli, it doesn't reflect on how good or bad a mother you are.

Fending off eating disorders

Many mothers are very aware of the dangers of eating disorders as increasing numbers of sufferers are reported in the media. As a result some women make a conscious effort never to mention dieting to their daughter. But that may not be enough to shelter her from these issues.

If mothers do diet or, as many women call it, 'just watching what I eat', children, particularly daughters, are likely to pick up on their weight concerns. Children will notice if you skip meals or say 'I shouldn't really' as you take another chocolate biscuit.

You can't completely shield them from the world of weight control, but if you are trying to lose weight, set them a good example by doing it sensibly through healthy eating.

Likewise, try not to worry about what other people think about your daughter's round tummy or your son's bony appearance. The most important thing is that your children are healthy and are developing a healthy relationship with food. So make sure they don't get the feeling that their appearance is somehow a disappointment to you.

The way forward is to separate your own negative food issues from your child's eating. Be careful not to be too controlling, as a child needs to rely on her own internal hunger and satiety cues. So don't restrict food excessively or coerce her to eat up. She also needs to be allowed to make some of her own decisions about what to eat so that she can learn how to make good choices and feel a sense of control.

Don't forget

O Your relationship with food inevitably affects the way you feed your child.

O By looking at the role food played in your own upbringing and your current feelings about eating and weight, you will be able to take a more objective view of your child's eating habits and any problems he may have.

O Thinking about your own relationship with food could also help you recognize how you could be negatively affecting your child's eating.

O Research has shown that women with eating disorders and those who have weight problems sometimes over-control their child's food intake. This can result in the child being unable to regulate her own eating.

O Try not to be too controlling over your child's diet. Give him some choices and let him enjoy treats sometimes.

O You don't need to resolve your own negative food issues to be able to promote healthy eating and a more positive approach to food in your child.

O Set realistic standards and try not to be too rigid about your own eating habits or your child's.

Healthy eating for your child's development

Eating patterns are set early in life. By helping your little ones to establish good dietary habits in childhood you will be preparing them to eat well for life. Healthy eating is not just about having the right mix of foods or nutrients; it is also about developing good dietary habits and a sensible attitude to food. In the short term a good diet will ensure your children get all the protein, iron, calcium and other nutrients that they need for healthy growth and development; in the long term it will reduce their risks of developing many major illnesses, including heart disease and some forms of cancer.

Most parents would agree that it's important to offer children a healthy mix of foods every day, but they might not aways know what that combination should be. However, once you are aware of the nutrition basics you will be much better equipped to pick your way through the shopping minefield and choose the 'right' stuff. And by the time you've finished reading this chapter you'll be less likely to accept that highly processed foods are as healthy as their manufacturers would have you believe.

As your child develops from a baby into a tweenie and beyond, her dietary needs will change. Babies need nutrient-dense meals and snacks as they are growing rapidly; however, from the age of two, children can very gradually start to have a diet with a bit less fat and more fibre. By the age of about five, they should be enjoying the kind of diet we think of as healthy for adults. As your child grows older you will have less influence over what she eats and she will have more meals away from home: at school, at friends' houses and at parties. By helping her to understand why it is important that she should eat well and by giving her the opportunity to make decisions about her what she eats, she'll be more likely to make healthy choices when you're not there.

While schools have some responsibility to teach children about nutrition, your child is only really going to take this information on board if you reinforce the messages at home and make healthy eating part of her everyday life.

First foods for babies (0–12 months)

Ideally babies should be breast-fed exclusively for the first six months of life, according to the World Health Organisation (WHO) and the UK's Department of Health. This recommendation is based on evidence that, for the majority of healthy full-term babies under six months old, breast milk is sufficient to meet all of their nutrient requirements, as well as offering many health benefits. Likewise, they recommend that neither breast-fed nor bottle-fed babies should receive any solids until they're six months old.

If you are breast-feeding your baby, it is still beneficial for your baby if you continue to feed in this way, even when you have started to introduce solids. The longer you can breast-feed, the greater the benefits for your baby.

All of the guidelines over the page apply to both bottle-fed and breast-fed babies.

Can't wait for solids?

If you feel that your baby is too hungry to wait until he reaches six months old before you introduce solids, try increasing the number of breast-feeds or the amount of formula you're giving him in order to sate his appetite. You might find that this is enough. If you do decide to wean a bit before six months it is very unlikely to cause any problems, but there may be benefits in waiting – especially if you have a family history of allergies. You should certainly wait until your baby is at least four months old: weaning any sooner than this is associated with particular health risks, including a greater incidence of eczema, wheezing and chest infections in childhood, and also with increases in body fat.

Starting solids

When you do start to wean your baby you should give him only foods suitable for his age (see pages 64–5). It is also important to make sure that all utensils are clean.

As the very first 'solid' food, baby rice mixed with a baby's normal milk (expressed breast milk or formula) usually goes down well. It doesn't taste much different from the milk he is used to and can be made fairly runny to begin with.

The key to weaning is to take things slowly: learning to handle solids and getting used to new flavours can take time. Some babies want more from day one, but it takes a while for the digestive system to adjust, so start with one very small meal (about two teaspoons). Later, you can give him more food as and when he wants it and build up to two then three meals a day.

Initially all foods should be puréed, then you can gradually make them less smooth. If you have waited until six months to begin weaning, you could start with purées and move on to coarser food after just a few weeks. If you start weaning earlier you can begin to introduce some lumps from six months. Your baby will let you know if you've made his food too lumpy before he's ready, usually by gagging. (If he seems to have a problem taking to lumps, see page 105 for more tips and advice.)

One of the easiest foods to use to introduce a bit of texture is banana. It's quite easy to mash with a fork and most babies like the taste. Once your baby has accepted this change to his diet you can start mashing most foods instead of puréeing, and give increasingly lumpy meals until he is eating chopped family meals – along with finger foods. This usually happens at around 12 months old, at which time solid foods will replace milk as the main part of his diet.

Offer food when your baby is not too tired or hungry – maybe halfway through a milk feed or, if he objects, after the feed. Heat one or two teaspoons of food thoroughly, allow it to cool and test the temperature before offering it to him.

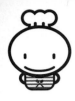

Widening the menu

When they start weaning babies don't need a very varied diet. However, over the next year or two you should encourage your child to eat a wider range of foods, as this helps him to develop a broader palate for later life.

To begin with try out new foods only at lunchtime, rather than in the evening. The reason for this is that it is easier to monitor your baby during waking hours in the unlikely event that he suffers some kind of reaction, and it is also a better time of day to seek out advice or medical help.

If you know that you have a family history of food allergies or intolerance, get advice from your health visitor or GP before you start weaning your baby.

How much and how often?

The number of meals, snacks and milk feeds a baby needs will vary with age, size, and other factors such as appetite and sleeping pattern. Generally, however, from about six to seven months onwards, babies will have three meals a day and two snacks. Most babies will also need about three breast-feeds or bottles during the course of the day: one when they wake, one mid-afternoon with a snack and one at bedtime. If they are still having feeds mid-morning and at lunchtime at this age these can gradually be phased out.

Around this time babies can also start having some finger foods (see the list on page 65). Most will enjoy chewing on something like a rice cake or toast finger, especially when they're teething. If you give them small round food though – such as a cherry tomato or grape – chop it in half to avoid any risk of choking and do not leave them unattended while they are eating.

As far as portion sizes are concerned, you can generally be guided by your baby's appetite. However, if he is underweight your health visitor may advise you to offer larger portions or to make meals more energy-dense; usually by using extra fat in cooking. If your baby is overweight, on the other hand, you may be advised to serve smaller portions or make meals less energy-dense by including more fruit and vegetables.

Never try to make your baby eat more than he wants. At the beginning, he is still getting most of the nourishment he needs from milk, and in the early days of weaning the aim is just to get him used to eating and enjoying solid food. It is also good to encourage self-feeding as soon as he is ready (see Chapter 1).

If your child has reflux (where milk is regurgitated back up into the oesophagus causing vomiting, heartburn, pain and discomfort) it can often be alleviated by weaning onto solids early. These can be easier to keep down, but make sure you talk to your GP or health visitor first.

Moving on to solids

Good first foods

○ Baby rice mixed with your baby's usual milk.

○ Stewed fruit, e.g. apple, pear.

○ Boiled or steamed vegetables, e.g. carrot, potato.

Foods to try only after six months

○ Meat, poultry and fish.

○ Beans or pulses such as lentils.

○ Full-fat milk in cooking, e.g. cheese sauce.

○ Full-fat dairy products, e.g. yoghurt, fromage frais, cheese.

○ Foods containing gluten, e.g. bread, Weetabix, pasta.

○ Cooked eggs.

○ Citrus fruit and fruit juice, e.g. orange.

Foods to avoid for the first year

○ Honey – this can very rarely cause infant botulism.

○ Salt – a baby's kidneys can't cope with lots of salt, so don't add any when cooking or at the table, and avoid salty foods like bacon, sausages or other processed foods.

○ Sugar – this provides calories without essential nutrients and can cause decay in newly emerging teeth.

○ Whole peanuts or other nuts. If you have a family history of allergies it is recommended that peanuts be avoided until at least three years of age.

○ Unpasteurized cheese.

○ Uncooked eggs.

Finger foods for 6-12 months

O Unsalted rice cakes.

O Baby breadsticks or fingers of wholemeal bread baked in the oven.

O Cooked vegetables, e.g. carrot sticks, green beans.

O Soft fruit, e.g. banana, pear or peach.

O Coarsely grated cheese.

Drinks

O When solids are first introduced, babies should still be given breast milk or 500–600ml of formula a day.

O Cow's milk should not be given to your baby as a drink for the first year.

O In addition to milk, the best drink is tap water (boiled and cooled until babies are six months old). It's a good idea to start offering water with each meal as soon as you start weaning; your baby probably won't take much to start with, but the amount they drink will gradually increase.

O Most babies don't need to drink anything other than milk and water. If you feel strongly that you want to give something else, or you are concerned that your baby may not be getting enough iron, you could give a cup of diluted orange juice with meals.

O Bottles shouldn't be used for sugary drinks – even fruit juice or baby drinks – as this increases the likelihood of tooth decay.

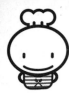

Feeding your growing toddler (1–2 years)

At this age, solids become more important in a child's diet and milk should no longer be the main source of nutrition. In fact, toddlers need only 300ml rather than 500–600ml of milk per day, and they can now be given full-fat cow's milk instead of breast-milk or formula. If you are still breast-feeding, two feeds a day should be sufficient alongside the dairy foods your baby will also be eating.

Meeting your toddler's dietary needs

You don't need to be concerned about limiting your toddler's fat intake. This doesn't mean that she can eat lots of fatty foods, like chips, but it does mean that you should give her full-fat milk and dairy products such as yoghurt and cheese. (Children shouldn't have semi-skimmed milk or any low-fat dairy products until they are at least two years old, and then only if they are eating well.)

A healthy diet for a toddler also differs from that required by an adult in that it contains fewer bulky, high-fibre foods. A toddler's stomach can't cope with foods such as wholemeal pasta and brown rice. A diet high in fibre will also make her feel full too quickly and can reduce the amount of iron and calcium she can absorb. However, it's still a good idea to offer her wholemeal rather than white bread, as toddlers do need some fibre. (And if they get used to eating white bread it can be very difficult to get them to change to wholemeal later.)

At this young age it is still important not to add salt and sugar to their foods; you might prefer saltier or sweeter food but toddlers don't, and they'll be better off when they are older if they don't get a taste for them now. Instead, you can start to cook food with a stronger flavour, if your child likes it, by using garlic, herbs and spices to add a bit of zest.

Toddlers are particularly vulnerable to iron deficiency, so it's important to ensure they get an adequate intake. This is done most easily by including some red meat in their diet: shepherd's pie or pasta bolognese are often successful choices, as some toddlers don't like the texture of proper pieces of meat and find them difficult to eat. If you are a vegetarian, there are also many good non-meat sources of iron which you should be sure to offer your child.

Eating foods rich in vitamin C alongside iron-rich ones will help increase the absorption of this important mineral (see page 83).

Many one-year-olds are fairly adventurous eaters, so serve them a wide range of foods while you can. In particular, offer different types of fruit and vegetables in order to get your children into the habit of eating them. And as well as serving vegetables within other dishes (such as in a pasta sauce), make sure your children are also given individual pieces of carrot, broccoli, and so on, so that they become familiar with the different tastes.

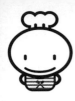

Snack time

Structure your toddler's eating throughout the day by serving three meals and incorporating two snacks. At this age, snacks still make up a substantial part of her diet because she can't eat enough at one meal to keep her going until the next. Appetites may also vary at mealtimes or disappear completely, so when it comes to snacks, make every mouthful count.

Snack times should be an opportunity for toddlers to catch up on any foods they might be missing out on at mealtimes – not a chance to have biscuits, cakes, sweets and crisps. Some toddlers need more at snack times than others, but you can expect them to eat something like a small banana or a half to one slice of bread. However, it is important not to give children the idea that if they don't like the meal they're given, they can have a biscuit later instead.

Bin the bottle

If your baby was bottle-fed rather than breast-fed, she should now be encouraged to switch from the bottle to a lidded cup. Likewise, if you stop breast-feeding when your baby is about a year old she can go straight to having milk from a cup. Water should also be given in a lidded cup.

Many one-year-olds are used to having a bottle at bedtime and find it very comforting. If this is the case, it's OK to continue with it if they are just drinking from the bottle before they are put into their cot, but bottles of milk should no longer be given throughout the rest of the day.

Water, water everywhere...

One- to two-year-olds who have milk from a bottle generally drink too much milk, which has a knock-on effect in that they may then be too full to eat the solids they require. Drinking fruit juice or squash from a bottle poses the same problem, as well as being a major cause of tooth decay. The best drink for toddlers between meals is water.

Nursery food for pre-schoolers (3-4 years)

With a few exceptions, three- and four-year-olds can eat more or less the same foods as adults, so there's no need to cook them special meals – just give them child-sized portions. However, there are some ways in which the pre-schooler's overall diet should differ from an adult's.

Although they may act like little grown-ups, pre-school-aged children are not quite ready for the low-fat, high-fibre diet that is recommended for us. Instead, their diet should gradually change so that they are eating an adult-style healthy diet by about five years old.

The milk they are drinking should still be semi-skimmed, as skimmed milk isn't suitable for children under five and, unless they're overweight, they still need a diet packed with energy-giving foods to meet all their requirements for

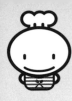
A toddler's diet should feature the following foods every day

O Milk and dairy products.

O Protein foods, such as meat, fish, eggs, beans and lentils.

O Starchy foods, such as bread, potatoes, pasta and rice.

O Fruit and vegetables.

Snacks

For the high chair

O Yoghurt.

O Pots of fruit purée.

O Breadsticks and vegetable batons with houmous.

On the go

O Breadsticks.

O A mini box of raisins.

O A banana.

O Rice cakes (without added salt).

O Pieces of fruit in a pot (such as apple, pear, satsuma, halved grapes).

O A cream cheese sandwich.

I want...

In the pre-school years, children are increasingly exposed to different types of food as they start going to nursery, play dates and parties. They are also likely to see food adverts on TV and notice packaged food in the shops that features their favourite characters. As a result, they may start to demand unhealthy foods, so you need to decide how much of it you're happy to let them eat (for example, one biscuit a day, crisps once a week) and stick to it.

growth and an active lifestyle. And, whatever their weight, pre-schoolers need plenty of vitamins and minerals to enable healthy development.

Like toddlers, pre-schoolers are also vulnerable to iron deficiency. Among four- to six-year-old children, 3 per cent of boys and 8 per cent of girls are anaemic, so a good intake of iron is essential, along with a high vitamin C intake to enhance its absorption (see pages 82-3).

Feeding schoolchildren (5–10 years)

As I mentioned earlier, once children reach five years old they should be having the type of diet we would consider healthy for an adult. So that means trying to encourage them to eat plenty of fruit and vegetables and to have a diet which is lower in fat and higher in fibre. While most parents have high ideals when they start feeding their child, these can sometimes slip when they get to school age.

A healthy diet for this age group includes:

O At least five portions of various fruit and vegetables a day.

O Lots of starchy foods, such as bread and pasta, including some high-fibre varieties every day.

O Moderate amounts of protein-rich foods such as meat, fish, eggs, beans and lentils. This should include two portions of fish a week, one of which should be oily, such as mackerel or salmon.

O Moderate amounts of low-fat dairy foods, including semi-skimmed or skimmed milk, yoghurt and cheese.

O Small amounts of fatty or sugary foods.

According to the Food Standards Agency, the selection of foods set out above should provide the ideal balance of nutrients when used as the basis of your child's diet.

Lessons in taste

Influences from outside the home increase as children reach school, so it becomes ever more important to teach them about healthy eating. At this age they are more likely to demand salty and sugary food and drinks. Children's main source of excess sugar is sweetened fizzy drinks, which contribute to weight problems and tooth decay, so it's really worth encouraging a tap-water habit early on (see page 112).

Most children consume more than twice the amount of salt they should. Processed foods are the main source, but salt in home cooking is also a problem and table salt is another culprit. Children who are allowed to add salt to their food have been found to have increased systolic blood pressure, so keep that salt cellar off the table.

School dinners and packed lunches

By the time your child is five, he will be having lunch at school most days. The TV chef Jamie Oliver has done a lot to raise awareness of the importance of healthy school meals and to highlight the poor quality of much of the food currently being served. As a result of his campaigning there has been some improvement in what is being offered, but you should still take time to investigate the menus at your child's school before deciding whether to give him school meals or packed lunches. If the meals aren't very good you can campaign for improvements, but it might be sensible to provide a packed lunch until the food gets better.

If you are making a packed lunch every day, keep the meals varied and get your child involved in planning what you pack – otherwise you may be giving him a well-balanced lunch that he doesn't like or isn't 'cool' amongst his peers, so it will be simply swapped or thrown in the bin. Some schools send home anything that isn't eaten, which can be very useful to show a parent what is working for their child, but that doesn't happen everywhere.

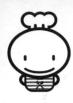

Bear in mind, too, that children are generally given a limited time for eating and there will also be many distractions. So keep lunches simple. You might find that satsumas are not eaten because a small child has trouble peeling them, or that food in tubs is left untouched because they cannot get the lid off. These problems are easily solved if you are aware of them – you can give the satsuma in a bag already peeled, get a tub with an easier lid, or ask the school if someone can help.

Snacks

For children of school age regular snacks between meals aren't as important as they are for younger children; in fact, most won't need a mid-morning snack if they've eaten a reasonable breakfast (see page 146 for difficult breakfast eaters). However, fruit can only be a good thing, so if this is offered as a snack at school they should be encouraged to have it.

Keep any after-school snacks small and healthy. If your children complain that they are starving, this is an ideal time to present them with a bowl of chopped fruit, such as pear or apple, or maybe some vegetable soup. If a healthy snack isn't enough to satisfy them, you could always serve their evening meal earlier than usual.

Fuelling physical activity

Children of school age generally become less active in their play and spend less time simply running around and more time watching TV or playing computer games. So to encourage a

Tips for healthy packed lunches

O Vary the type of bread in sandwiches, for example: whole-meal pitta, wraps, granary rolls and oatcakes. Or try pasta or rice salad for a change.

O Use different fillings, for example: ham, cheese, egg, chicken, houmous, tuna.

O Add a bit of salad to sandwiches or put cherry tomatoes, carrot sticks, and so on, in the lunch box.

O Give fruit that is quick and easy to eat, such as grapes, bananas, fruit salad or pineapple chunks in a pot, or dried fruit – e.g. raisins or apricots.

O Keep treats healthy. Instead of a chocolate biscuit, offer a mini fruit scone or bun, malt loaf, cereal and fruit bars, or homemade banana or carrot cake.

O Beware of pre-packed foods advertised as suitable for lunch boxes. Many are high in salt, saturated fat or sugar and they can be expensive. It's usually possible to give a healthier and cheaper alternative, such as oat cakes with slices of Cheddar, or natural yoghurt with some fruit on the top.

O For extra tips and a fortnight of new packed-lunch ideas see www.food.gov.uk.

healthy lifestyle and reduce the chances of a weight problem, the right diet should be accompanied by a greater focus on physical activity (see page 211).

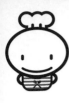

Get the nutrition know-how

Understanding the basics of good nutrition can help you and your child appreciate the importance of eating certain types of foods and enable you to make healthier choices. A child as young as three can already begin to understand that, for example, milk has calcium in it, which is good for bones and teeth.

Use the table of nutrition facts for kids (on pages 84–7) to help explain to your children what different foods do for the body. This information will help them to understand why they need more of some foods but less of others, and why you are encouraging a certain kind of diet. As your children get older they may want more detailed information about certain foods or particular nutrients.

Teach children about nutrition when you're both relaxed, NOT at the table when they're refusing to eat their vegetables.

Here's the low-down on all the key elements of diet – and how much or how little of each is good for your child.

Energy

Calories (Kcal) are simply the unit used to measure energy: so if a food gives you lots of energy, it will also contain lots of calories. If more calories are consumed than are needed, the excess is stored as fat.

Children have three sources of energy: carbohydrates, protein and fat. Parents often have a fourth one, too: alcohol.

Carbohydrates

The main source of energy in our diet. Carbohydrates can be divided into starches and sugars.

Starches, also called complex carbohydrates, include potatoes, rice, pasta, cous cous, bread and breakfast cereals. Unrefined starches such as wholemeal bread and brown rice contain more vitamins, minerals and fibre than processed foods, such as white bread and white rice. Intakes of unrefined starches should gradually be increased between the ages of about two and five years.

Sugars occur naturally in fruit where they are accompanied by other nutrients, such as vitamins A and C and potassium. Refined sugar, including white or brown sugar, syrup and honey provide calories but no other nutrients (known as empty calories). So sugary foods such as sweets and fizzy drinks should be consumed only in limited amounts. They also cause tooth decay, so they should be avoided between meals.

Protein

Needed for growth and development, protein is also required for building muscle tissue and helping the body repair itself. Protein deficiency is rarely a problem. In fact average preschoolers consume more than twice as much as they need, but there is no benefit in having extra protein: it doesn't make children grow taller, more muscular or stronger.

The best sources of protein are lean meat, fish, eggs, beans and lentils, as these provide other beneficial nutrients as well.

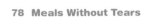

Products such as sausages, burgers and meat pies also provide protein, but they have high levels of saturated fat and salt too, so they are best eaten no more than once or twice a week.

Fat

A concentrated source of energy, fat provides more than twice the calories of carbohydrate, gram for gram.

Fats are necessary for the absorption of fat-soluble vitamins (A, D, E and K) and some fatty acids are vital for life. Both omega 3 and omega 6 fatty acids, found in vegetable oils such as sunflower and corn oils and in oily fish such as salmon, are essential nutrients and are good for the heart. Also, the omega 3 fatty acids from oily fish include EPA (eicosapentaenoic acid) and DHA (docosahexaenoic acid), which are important in brain development.

Monounsaturated fats, found in high levels in olive and rapeseed oils, are also considered healthy, as they are good for the heart.

Saturated fat, however, is regarded as unhealthy as high intakes of it can raise blood cholesterol levels and increase the risk of heart disease. Saturated fat is found primarily in meat, milk and dairy products such as cheese.

Trans-fats, used widely in foods such as biscuits and cakes, are now believed to be even more damaging to our health than saturated fats. Many countries restrict the use of trans-fats, a practice that is now starting to be adopted by some British supermarkets.

Oily Fish and omega 3

It is recommended that children of all ages eat at least two portions of fish a week, one of which should be oily. Oily fish such as salmon, mackerel and sardines contain lots of omega 3 fatty acids, which are important for brain development and have been linked with improved cognitive performance.

There are also plenty of expensive food products available with added omega 3, but oily fish is still the best source, and it contains protein, iron and vitamins A and D too.

Fibre

Two types of fibre should feature in our diet: insoluble and soluble.

Insoluble fibre is what we think of as roughage; it helps food move though the digestive system. This fibre is found in wholegrain cereals, wholemeal bread, beans, fruit and vegetables. Children who don't have enough are more likely to get constipated, although an adequate fluid intake is also important to prevent this happening. In the long term, a diet with plenty of fibre protects against certain diseases of the bowel.

Soluble fibre is found in oats, beans and lentils. This form of fibre helps reduce blood cholesterol levels and is useful in controlling blood sugar levels.

A high-fibre diet increases satiety, which can be a problem for very small children as they feel full before they've

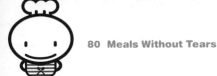

consumed enough calories and nutrients. For older children who are overweight, however, adding more fibre to the diet can be beneficial.

Water

It is often forgotten, but water is an essential nutrient. Every cell and tissue in the body requires water. Fluids are needed to carry oxygen and nutrients around the body and also to remove waste.

Children should have water regularly throughout the day: aim for a cup or glass of fluid with each meal and snack. Dehydration can result in headaches and listlessness, and it also contributes to constipation. Urine colour will give you a good indication of whether your little ones are getting enough water: if it is dark yellow, rather than pale, they need to drink more.

Vitamin A

This vitamin is required for good vision, and is particularly important for enabling eyes to adapt to dim light. Vitamin A is also needed to produce healthy skin cells and to support a good immune system.

There are two forms of vitamin A found in food: retinol, which is present in liver, oily fish and dairy products; and beta-carotene (pro-vitamin A), which is found in carrots, pumpkin, apricots and cantaloupe melons.

B vitamins

There are several B vitamins found in food, all of which are important for different reasons:

Thiamin (B$_1$) is needed to release energy from foods, especially from carbohydrates, and to promote a healthy nervous system. It is found in wholegrain and fortified cereals, salmon, tuna, peas, beans and nuts.

Riboflavin (B$_2$) is also required to help release energy from foods. Dairy foods, eggs and meat are the best sources.

Niacin is required for many of the chemical reactions taking place in the body, especially those for energy production. It is generally found in high-protein foods such as meat, fish, dairy products and pulses.

Pantothenic acid helps convert food to energy and produce neurotransmitters and haemoglobin. It is in many foods, including chicken, oats, egg yolks and broccoli.

Folic acid is needed for making DNA for new cells. Sources include most breakfast cereals, oranges and leafy green vegetables.

Vitamin B$_6$ helps the body use protein and fats. It is found in nuts, meat, fish and beans.

Vitamin B$_{12}$ is needed to make new cells. It is found naturally only in animal foods (meat, fish, eggs, dairy foods) but is added to many cereals and vegetarian foods.

Vitamin C

This vitamin is important in the healing of wounds, a strong immune system and to increase iron absorption. The best sources are citrus fruits such as oranges, strawberries and other berries, kiwi fruit, potatoes, broccoli, cauliflower and leafy green vegetables.

Vitamin D

Vitamin D is responsible for controlling the body's absorption of calcium. We get most of what we need from the action of ultra violet light on our skin. However, in northern latitudes people don't always have enough exposure to sunlight, so dietary sources such as eggs, dairy products, butter, margarine and oily fish become essential, particularly in winter.

Vitamin E

Acting as an antioxidant – along with beta-carotene, vitamin C and selenium – vitamin E reduces damage to cells in the body caused by free-radicals and decreases the risk of cancer and heart disease. Vegetable oils (particularly sunflower), nuts, wholemeal cereals and leafy vegetables are all good sources.

Vitamin K

Proteins involved in the blood-clotting system require vitamin K. Leafy green vegetables are the best source, but other vegetables also contain significant amounts, as do fruits, cereals, meat, milk and margarine.

Calcium

Calcium is vital for the healthy formation of bones and teeth, and is also needed for blood clotting and muscle contraction. Dairy products are the most important source for children, but other sources of calcium include fish, leafy green vegetables, sunflower and sesame seeds and almonds. Fish with edible bones such as sardines are a particularly good source.

Iron

Required for healthy red blood cells, which carry oxygen around the body, iron is absorbed more readily from meat and fish than from non-meat sources. Fortified breakfast cereals can be a valuable source of iron, but read the packaging carefully as some cereals, including all organic varieties, don't have iron added. Other non-meat sources of iron include chickpeas, leafy green vegetables and dried fruit.

Having a good dose of vitamin C alongside iron in a meal can more than double the absorption of iron from non-animal sources. For example, have some diluted orange juice with breakfast cereal; broccoli and cauliflower with chickpea curry; or strawberries after a sandwich.

Potassium

Potassium is important in regulating the fluid balance within the body and to help muscles to work efficiently. High intakes of this mineral can help balance out the harmful effects of too much salt and are linked with lower blood pressure. Good

Nutrition facts for kids

What's it called?	Where is it found?
Energy (calories)	All food and drink, except water
Carbohydrates	Starches: bread, pasta, potatoes, cereals, rice and yams Sugary foods: sweets, biscuits, cakes and regular fizzy drinks
Protein	Meat, fish, milk, eggs, cheese, yoghurt, beans, lentils
Fats	Oily fish: salmon, sardines, mackerel, fresh tuna and trout Butter, margarine, chips, crisps, biscuits, cakes, sausages, burgers
Fibre	Wholemeal bread, brown rice, brown pasta and brown breakfast cereals, fruit, vegetables
Water	It's good to drink plain tap water. You also get water from food like juicy pears, tomatoes and soup

Why do I need it?

To grow and to move around. Eating is like putting petrol in a car; however, if you eat more than you need, it is stored and you can become overweight.

For energy so you can run around and play.
Starches provide energy to keep you going for a long time. Brown bread and pasta, etc., will give you vitamins, minerals and fibre too. **Sugary foods** taste nice but don't make you healthy. They also cause tooth decay.

To make you grow and have strong muscles.

They give you energy, and some foods, such as oily fish, contain omega 3 fats, which are good for your brain.
Too much unhealthy fat (saturated and trans-fats) is bad for your heart.

It helps the food move through your body. If you don't have enough, it can be difficult to poo.

To move nutrients around the body and clean your insides. It also helps keep you cool. If you don't have enough, you can get headaches and bad moods, or have trouble pooing.

What's it called?	Where is it found?
Vitamin A	Carrots, pumpkins, apricots, eggs, fish
B vitamins	Broccoli, breakfast cereals, meat, milk, fish
Vitamin C	Oranges, kiwi fruit, strawberries, broccoli, potatoes
Vitamin D	Egg yolk, dairy products, oily fish. We get most of our vitamin D from sunlight on our skin
Vitamin E	Sunflower oil, nuts, leafy green vegetables
Vitamin K	Leafy green vegetables, Brussels sprouts, milk, margarine
Calcium	Milk, cheese, yoghurt, sardines
Iron	Meat, fish, some breakfast cereals, dried apricots
Potassium	Potatoes, bananas and other fruit
Sodium	Salt, crisps, bacon, ready-meals

Why do I need it?
To help you see well in the dark.

So your body can change the food you eat into energy you can use.

So that your skin will heal when you get hurt.

To help make your bones grow strong.

To keep all the cells in your body healthy, including your skin.

It makes your blood clot when you have a cut or graze, so that blood doesn't keep pouring out.

To build strong bones and teeth.

A metal that makes it possible for your blood to carry oxygen all around your body. It also gives blood its red colour.

So that your muscles can work well.

A tiny bit keeps you healthy; too much is bad for the heart.

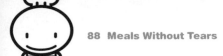

sources include most fruit and vegetables, but bananas and potatoes in particular.

Sodium

Sodium is required to control the retention of fluid in the body. Most people, including children, take in too much sodium in the form of salt. Excess sodium is excreted, but as this happens it pulls fluid from the body's cells, leading to high blood pressure. Lots of the salt in children's diets comes from processed foods such as breakfast cereals, sausages, burgers, chicken nuggets, ready-made meals and sauces and savoury snacks such as crisps.

The maximum amount of salt children should be having varies with age:

Age	Daily intake should be no more than
Under 12 months	1g
1–3 years	2g
4–6 years	3g
7–10 years	5g

See Chapter 9 for lots of ideas on fun ways to teach your children about nutrition, and get them involved in learning how to make healthy food choices.

How to read food labels

Many foods aimed at children have some sort of health claim, but it's the things they don't advertise that you need to be most wary about. Sweets bearing the slogan 'contains real fruit juice' can still be more than 90 per cent sugar, while a kid's cheese product that is advertised as a good source of calcium probably won't carry a warning that it is saltier than seawater. A survey by the Food Commission found that only 1 in 10 products aimed specifically at children could be regarded as healthy – and the study didn't even include obvious junk foods such as crisps, soft drinks or confectionery.

The bottom line is that you shouldn't trust any food claims until you have looked at the small print. And that means the nutritional information panel and list of ingredients. Many products now carry colour-coded information on the front of packs too, which can be useful for quickly comparing products when you're shopping.

However, bear in mind that the dietary information on food products is usually judged on the basis of adult recommendations: so a six-year-old could eat a pre-packed sandwich containing 2g salt, and although this might show an amber traffic light for medium, and therefore be considered as not that unhealthy, it actually contains two thirds of the daily maximum amount recommended for her age group.

The table on the next page will help you to establish whether a food contains an unhealthy amount of fat, sugar and salt.

How to read food labels

	Amount per 100g	
	A lot (g)	A little (g)
Total fat	20	3
Saturated fat	5	1
Sugar	10	2
Labelled as 'carbohydrates (of which sugar)'		
Salt	1.25	0.25
Sodium (multiply by 2.5 to get salt value)	0.5	0.1

Source: Food Standards Agency

Be wary of any products with added vitamins, minerals, omega 3 fatty acids, probiotics, prebiotics or other 'healthy' additives. These are often used to enhance the appeal of otherwise unhealthy products, so don't buy them just for the added ingredients. Sugary drinks fortified with vitamin C and white bread with added omega 3 are no substitute for fruit and vegetables or oily fish.

Help your child to look more closely at food labels, rather than just focusing on the pictures on packs or the free toys. Chapter 9 has some ideas to help you do this.

It is best to avoid regularly giving children foods in which the following items appear in the list of ingredients:

○ Hydrogenated or partially hydrogenated fat or vegetable oil. These contain unhealthy trans-fats.

○ Lots of added sugar. And bear in mind that sugar comes in many guises: sucrose, glucose, fructose, maltose, dextrose, inverted sugar, hydrolysed starch, corn syrup, glucose syrup, and so on. These forms of sugar provide calories but no beneficial nutrients. Products sweetened with concentrated apple or grape juice appear to be a healthier option, but don't be fooled into thinking that they are a substitute for fruit: they encourage children to develop a taste for sugar instead of fruit while lacking any fibre.

○ A long list of additives. Foods with lots of colours, flavourings, flavour enhancers, stabilizers, and so on, are usually over-processed and contain too much fat, salt or sugar.

○ Artificial sweeteners. These are not allowed in food or drink aimed at children under three years and many campaigners believe they should be banned from all children's products.

Junk food – a little of what they fancy

Children will inevitably be drawn to junk food. Even if you never give them burgers, crisps, chocolate or cola at home, they will be served them at other people's houses and parties. Nor can you stop them taking an interest in junk food when it's advertised on TV, pictured in the windows of fast-food restaurants in the high street and attractively packaged in the shops. They

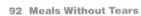

might hear friends talking about trips to fast-food restaurants too and this can have a big effect on them as they get older.

Even if you hate the idea of your child eating certain foods, don't ban them altogether: if you do this, it may backfire. Banning sweets, for example, implies they are special and different from other foods, and thus more interesting and desirable. So when your child does get access to them, at a party or friend's house or when he has pocket money to spend, he might be more inclined to eat as many as he can.

It is much better to tell your children that different foods do different things for your body, so you need them in varying amounts. For example, 'Milk helps your bones to grow strong, so you need to drink some every day;' 'Sweets taste nice, but they don't make you strong or healthy, so you should have them only occasionally.' Try to focus on the positive and emphasize how nice some of the more desirable foods are, such as juicy strawberries or fresh pineapple. Find healthier alternatives for many of the foods they might like, too – you can make your own popcorn without any added salt, or cook healthier versions of foods such as burgers or chicken nuggets.

A little of what they fancy does no harm, as long as they're getting a lot of what they need.

Decide the limits you're happy with for foods such as sweets, crisps and biscuits, for example, and whether your children are allowed them once a day or once a week. There is a number

Parties and special occasions

When it comes to children's parties, days out and special occasions, you may be better off accepting that they are going to eat badly and let them enjoy it. Also, it can be good for children to have the opportunity to experience new foods: it's all part of the learning process. However, if they go to a party at lunchtime, don't take the attitude that as healthy eating is out the window for the whole day, anything goes. Instead plan a more nutritious supper later to balance out their intake.

of ways you can do this: you could perhaps say they can have sweets only on a Saturday afternoon; or once a week and let them choose the time and day. Another way of limiting intake, which could work for older children, is to give them a tub containing the week's allowance of junk food – for instance a packet of crisps, some chocolate and a few sweets – and give them the choice and responsibility for when they eat them.

A balanced diet doesn't have to be implemented religiously on a daily basis, so don't feel guilty and don't make your children feel guilty for enjoying treats. Cakes, chocolate and so on all have a place in a balanced diet. However, do make sure that the 'special occasions' on which certain less healthy foods are allowed do not become every time you're with friends, all weekend and the entire school holidays.

Don't forget

O Children's nutrient requirements change as they get older. Babies need plenty of fat and foods which are energy-dense, but by the age of five years children should be having a diet lower in fat and higher in fibre.

O Children tend to eat away from home more often as they get older. If your child takes a packed lunch to school, get her involved in planning a balanced meal that she would like to eat.

O Teach your child the basics of nutrition and encourage him to take responsibility for choosing a good balance of foods to keep his body healthy.

O If you learn how to read food labels better, it will be easier to make good food choices.

O Don't ban certain foods or display a disapproving attitude towards them – this will just make them appear more attractive. Also remind your child that there are no bad foods, just foods she should eat less often.

O Rather than focusing too much on unhealthy junk foods, emphasize the positives and encourage a love of healthier, yet still tasty, alternatives.

Fussy eating and limited diets

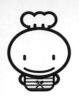

We are all fussy eaters to some extent: no doubt there are certain foods you don't eat. Most of us would prefer our children to have a more varied diet than they do, but we can't expect them to eat everything they're served. So first of all you should ask yourself whether your child's fussy eating is really a problem for them, or just for you.

How does fussy eating affect the growing child?

If your child's diet is limited and results in him missing out on entire food groups, there could be health implications. Refusing milk and dairy products could result in weaker bones; not eating fruit or vegetables increases the risk of asthma and iron deficiency in childhood and can increase the risk of heart disease and certain cancers in the long term. It can also be a problem if your child refuses to eat meals with lumps, runny foods or anything that hasn't come from a jar, as this obviously limits his food choices.

In this chapter I explain the possible consequences of refusing particular types of food, and I give you some action plans to help you get your children to enjoy a more balanced diet.

If your child is not missing out whole food groups completely but is simply eating a very small range of foods, it may not actually be that bad for him, nutritionally; just irritating for you. If children are growing and developing well, have plenty of energy and are generally healthy and happy, they're unlikely to have any nutrient deficiencies.

If you still find it hard not to worry, think of 'Jam Boy' who hit the headlines in 2004. At the age of 15, he had suffered no obvious ill effects despite eating little more than jam sandwiches and milk from the age of four. That said, your child is more likely to get the nutrients he needs if he eats a wide range of foods.

General reasons for fussy eating

Children who eat well as babies often become pickier when they turn into toddlers. As they become increasingly independent they may refuse to eat certain foods as a way of asserting their newfound autonomy and of establishing some control. The key to surviving this irritation is not to rise to the bait. Your child may not really dislike a particular food, but if you make a fuss she's more likely to dig her heels in. So backing off at this stage can prevent a minor issue turning into a larger problem.

Remember too that picky eating may just be a way to get attention at mealtimes. It may get her negative attention, but for some that's better than no attention at all. She may also enjoy seeing that you show concern for her well-being, particularly if you start offering her other foods instead.

Unfortunately these mealtime battles are not just limited to the toddler years. Refusing food can continue to be a way of demonstrating independence or getting attention throughout childhood. Kids quickly realize there's very little you can do to make them eat, although we parents may take longer to recognize this. We want them to become independent and make good decisions, but it is difficult to allow them the space they need when we are worrying about the health implications of their choices.

Don't focus on what they won't eat – talk about what they will and be sure to praise healthy choices. For example, 'It's good you're eating cheese because it makes your bones strong.'

However, children are generally not being fussy over food just to annoy you; they may genuinely find certain flavours or textures of food unpleasant. It may also be that they are sensitive about other things too, such as itchy shirts, loud noises or strong smells, or that they like routine and predictability. It is just the way they are.

It can be particularly hard for parents to handle sudden changes in taste. A child might hate rice today even though it was his favourite food yesterday. This can be infuriating as he is unlikely to mention it until dinner is on the table. But try to be patient: he may be in a bad mood, or not particularly hungry, or just bored with having rice too often. Whatever the reason, making a big deal of it isn't going to help.

Fussy forever?

The good news is that fussy eating is often a temporary problem, and one that is much more common in pre-schoolers
than in older kids. An American study following children from
the ages of three to seven found that 70 per cent of them
were picky eaters at some stage, but only 10 per cent for the
entire period. Of course, 10 per cent is still significant and re-
flects the fact that, unfortunately, some children will always
be fussy about their food.

Children who won't try anything new

Children who are unwilling to try new foods are described as
neophobic. Some experts believe that this behaviour stems
from our ancestors, for whom it evolved so that they could
avoid eating anything poisonous. But since you are unlikely
to be giving your child anything toxic, this attitude can be
frustrating.

Neophobic children have been found to eat less fruit and
vegetables than their peers, and less protein foods, such
as meat. Some kids will say they don't like something even
before you put their plate down. They will refuse to taste it and
may even demand you remove the offending item. After such
a performance, many parents won't give their child the same

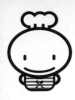
food again. They may try something else new or, more likely, go back to old favourites. Others will have one or two more attempts, but then accept that the child doesn't like it.

However, perseverance really is the key. Research has shown that children are more likely to accept a food if they are offered it on 10 to 15 occasions. So it is worth sticking at it.

Action plan

○ Be prepared to serve a new food up to 20 times before accepting that your child really doesn't like it.

○ Try only one new food per meal.

○ Give children new foods alongside ones they like.

○ Allow children to play with a new food: it helps them to become familiar with it and makes them more likely to try it.

○ Make sure they see you and other children eating new foods. They will then be more willing to do the same.

○ Don't force them to eat anything. You could insist they try one mouthful or add a star to a reward chart, but if they put up a lot of resistance, it may not be worth the battle. Some parents let their child spit out the mouthful if they don't like it – knowing they can do this can help a child get over her initial fear.

○ Praise your child for trying something new.

Dos and don'ts for handling fussy eaters

By learning how to handle fussy eaters you are more likely to be able to improve their diet and at the same time make mealtimes more enjoyable for everyone.

Do

○ Relax and take a step back. Sitting down to a meal shouldn't be a strain, so try to help your child develop a sense of pleasure in eating.

○ Remember: carrots work better than sticks – even with kids who hate vegetables! So give praise for tasting different foods, try a star chart or give a small (non-food) reward, such as a sticker, when they eat well at a meal.

○ Give them a few choices, but make all the options healthy.

○ Teach children about why they need different foods, but don't do this at the table when they're refusing to eat something. Help them to think about what foods their body needs in order to encourage them to take responsibility for looking after their body and keeping it healthy.

○ Get them involved in planning meals, shopping for food and cooking.

○ Serve a wide variety of foods on a regular basis. They may eat very few at first, but if you keep doing it you might be pleasantly surprised.

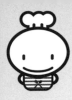

⊙ Be a good role model. Let your child see you eating and enjoying lots of different foods.

⊙ Even if you don't eat with your child, sit down with him and at least have a drink and relax.

⊙ Be positive. As a starting point, think about what she will eat, not what she won't. If your child is old enough (at least four or five years old), draw up three lists of food with her:

1 Foods she likes and is happy to eat.

2 Foods she hates (individual foods, not whole groups such as vegetables).

3 Foods she would be willing to try.

Do this when you are both relaxed and not rushed.

⊙ Try giving foods in different settings, such as on a picnic. If the dinner table has become a battleground more relaxed surroundings may help.

⊙ Write a list of 5–10 targets you'd like to achieve. Number one might be 'taste one vegetable'. Other targets could be 'eat one tablespoon of vegetables' or 'eat two different types of vegetables'. If your final goal is 'eat any type of vegetable and have three portions every day' you may never reach it, but by setting a series of targets you'll be able to see you're getting somewhere and mealtimes should be less fraught.

⊙ Talk to other parents – you are not alone.

Don't

○ Force a child to eat anything.

○ Nag at meals or hover over him as he eats. Children will pick up on your tension even if you say nothing.

○ Supervize each mouthful, for example – to ensure vegetables are eaten as well as sausages.

○ Offer food rewards for eating something, such as sweets for finishing carrots.

○ Withhold pudding if your child won't eat something. This just tells her one food is undesirable but the other is tasty.

○ Offer unhealthy alternatives or extra snacks if he doesn't eat the food served.

○ Assume your child won't eat certain foods at nursery or with friends just because she doesn't eat them at home. Peer pressure can work wonders on fussy eaters.

○ Label your child as a fussy eater and discuss the problem in front of him. This can simply reinforce the idea in his mind and lets him say, 'but you know I don't eat vegetables'.

○ Expect a complete turn-around overnight.

○ Give up if it seems slow going. Over time your child's diet should improve.

Jars of baby food – just delicious

You'd think anyone would prefer home cooking to a meal from a jar, but with babies this isn't always the case. You might feel quite insulted as your little one turns his nose up at your lovingly prepared dishes, then licks his lips as you produce a jar from the cupboard, but it's not uncommon behaviour.

Babies who regularly eat food from jars can find it hard to make the transition to freshly prepared foods. Others may decide they prefer the taste even though they've had them only occasionally. Both the texture and the taste of food from jars are different from those of home cooking, mainly because of the high temperatures used in its manufacture. If your baby is around a year old he will also be more suspicious of anything new, which can make the problem worse.

Nutritionally there is nothing wrong with eating baby food from jars. Strict rules control the content of food manufactured for children under three years old, which ensures that jars of baby food have an appropriate nutrient content and that no salt is added, as well as prohibiting the use of most additives and ensuring pesticide levels are carefully monitored. However, the sooner a child gets a taste for fresh food, the better.

The danger of a fondness for food in jars is that your baby could develop a liking for processed foods, and those manufactured for older children and adults generally contain unhealthy levels of salt, sugar and saturated fat.

Action plan

○ Give some homemade food at the beginning of a meal when your baby is hungriest, even if you give food from a jar afterwards. The more he eats your freshly prepared food, the more he will come to accept it.

○ Try mixing a bit of homemade food with food from a jar. Gradually adjust the proportions so that your child is eating more freshly prepared food, then stop giving him anything from a jar at all.

○ If your baby isn't having many finger foods, increase the range. This is a good way of introducing new textures and flavours. Include foods such as toast, sliced fruit, cooked vegetables, cheese and chicken to give a good variety.

○ Let your child see other children eating different foods.

○ If you're brave you could make your baby go cold turkey and simply stop serving him any food from jars. Rather than starve, he will eventually eat freshly prepared foods. It could be a quicker solution, but it might be more traumatic for you both!

No lumps, please!

Some babies are fine at the start of weaning but kick up a fuss later. They enjoy baby rice and puréed fruit and vegetables to begin with, but when you try to give them anything except the smoothest purée they seem to gag and choke or spit out their food. They may even vomit at the smallest hint of a lump. Babies or toddlers may refuse lumps simply because they're

not used to them. Research suggests that early introduction may be the key, and from six months babies can be given meals with a bit of texture. Babies who don't have any lumpy solids before 10 months have been found to be more likely to have feeding problems.

However, some babies never really take to lumpy dishes. They move from having just purées on to a combination of purées and finger foods, then to having their entire meal as pieces of food they can pick up with their fingers.

Action plan

O Gradually make baby food coarser by not puréeing it quite so much. If you have a hand-held blender, it's very easy to control the consistency of meals. Eventually you should be able simply to mash foods rather than using a liquidizer or blender. If your baby is used to eating only jars of food, add some slightly textured homemade food to a jar you know she likes.

O For now, avoid foods which are smooth with the odd lump, such as yoghurt with bits of fruit, or jars of pasta that have a smooth sauce with pieces of spaghetti.

O Introduce finger foods such as rice cakes or toast. Babies often find them more acceptable than lumps, despite their solid texture, and even those babies without teeth can gum them quite effectively. They may also be happy to dip these into mixed dishes or foods such as houmous or cream cheese.

O Gradually expand the range of finger foods eaten to include cheese, pieces of vegetable or fruit, and bits of chicken.

Nothing mushed or runny for me

Sometimes babies refuse baby food and will accept only foods they can pick up and eat themselves, such as toast, biscuits and bananas. Older children may also refuse mushy or runny foods, such as stews, sauces or yoghurt, and instead stick to solid ones, such as sandwiches, biscuits, crackers and chips.

With a baby it may simply be because he has a fierce sense of independence, but can't use a spoon efficiently. For older children it can be that they dislike the texture or the mess that accompany certain foods. Perhaps an over-anxious parent has attacked them with a cloth once too often. This can send the message that it's bad to get food on your face or anywhere else and may lead to a phobia for messy food.

Action plan

For a baby:

○ Allow him to eat any food with his fingers, for example, pasta, pieces of potato. Try not to worry about the mess until the meal is over (see page 157 for dealing with messy eaters).

○ Serve a wide variety of finger foods:

- ◉ Unsalted bread sticks, toast fingers, oatcakes or slices of pitta bread
- ◉ Cubes of cheese
- ◉ Slices of fruit, for example, apple, pear
- ◉ Cooked vegetables, e.g. peas, carrot sticks, green beans
- ◉ Pieces of chicken or fish

- Give him foods such as houmous, yoghurt or fruit purée to dip finger foods in.
- Help him to learn to use a spoon, although he's unlikely to be capable of spoon-feeding himself a whole meal if he's under the age of 18 months.
- If he doesn't object, sneak in a few spoonfuls of food, for example, some fish pie while he's busy trying to pick up peas.

For an older child:

- Enjoy some messy play together, for example, finger painting or sand.
- Encourage him to have fun and get messy with food sometimes. You could try making a pudding with layers of yoghurt and fruit compote or an ice-cream sundae.
- Let him see you get a bit messy without appearing worried and encourage him to do the same. You could both lick your fingers too.
- Be silly and eat some yoghurt with your finger.
- Keep cloths and wet wipes out of sight until he has finished eating.

No milk today – I hate it!

Milk is seen as a pure and natural foodstuff and vital for growing children, so it can be a worry if your little one refuses to drink it.

Sometimes when babies stop being breast-fed, they won't drink milk from a bottle or a cup, but this is usually only a temporary situation; once they realize breast milk isn't available they're likely gradually to increase the amount of milk they'll drink. Moving a toddler from a bottle on to a cup can result in similar problems, but these will also gradually improve with time.

Occasionally children dislike milk because it gives them cramps or makes them feel bloated and windy. This can be due to lactose intolerance, which means the child doesn't produce enough lactase (an enzyme which breaks down the lactose sugar in milk).

More rarely children with similar symptoms may be allergic to milk. Eczema, asthma, a runny nose and fatigue are additional indicators of an allergy. If you think your child may be having some kind of reaction to drinking milk, it's important to see your doctor for a proper diagnosis.

However, such physical reactions are rare. The most common reason for refusing milk is simply that a child doesn't like the taste.

Why is milk important?

Milk provides calcium and vitamin D, which are essential for strong bones. Children who don't drink it have been found to have weaker bones and increased risks of fracture and osteoporosis when they are older. Milk is also a good source of protein, iodine, magnesium, potassium and vitamins A and B_{12}.

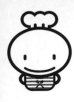

How much do they need?

Babies under 12 months who are not breast-fed need about 500 to 600 ml of milk per day. This doesn't all need to be taken as a drink. Some can be given on cereal or with other food and some in the form of yoghurt and other dairy foods.

The daily requirement for milk decreases to 300ml for one- to three-year-olds and older children should aim to have about three portions of dairy foods each day, including milk, yoghurt and cheese.

Action plan

O For babies recently weaned from breast milk, keep on offering formula or, if the baby is over 12 months, cow's milk. You could try different bottles or feeding cups.

O If your child rejects warm milk, try it cold, and vice versa.

O Try other milky drinks (in a cup, not a bottle):

⊙ Cocoa (with no or very little sugar)

⊙ Milkshake (blend a banana or strawberries with milk)

⊙ Lassi (blend milk, yoghurt and fruit)

O Add milk to other food:

⊙ Cereal (a Weetabix soaks up about 100ml milk if left for a few minutes)

⊙ Mashed potato

⊙ Any mushed baby food, such as pasta or shepherd's pie

⊙ White sauce or cheese sauce

⊙ Dessert, for example, rice pudding, custard

○ Serve more dairy foods; then it's fine to have less straight milk. The following have about the same amount of calcium as 100ml of milk:

- ⊙ Yoghurt (80g pot)
- ⊙ Cheese (20g piece)
- ⊙ Cream cheese (100g)

○ Give them other calcium-rich foods. The following have the same amount of calcium as 100ml milk:

- ⊙ Sardines (25g mashed with bones)
- ⊙ Dried figs (50g)
- ⊙ Curly kale (80g)
- ⊙ Tofu (25g)
- ⊙ Other soya products (Ask a doctor before giving soya milk to babies)

(N.B. It is difficult to get enough calcium from non-dairy foods, because there are not enough calcium-rich foods that children are willing to eat on a daily basis. Also the body absorbs calcium much more easily from dairy foods. So this is only a partial solution.)

○ Tell older children why they need milk and dairy foods, then work out a solution together.

○ If you think they're still not getting enough calcium, talk to your doctor or health visitor. They may advise supplements.

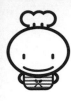

You can lead a baby to water...

Children refusing to drink water is a common problem. At the start of weaning, babies often drink very little water, perhaps just a few sips. This is partly because they're not used to it and also because most of their diet is in the form of milk, so they don't need a lot of additional fluid at this stage.

However, parents often think their baby doesn't like water before she has had a proper chance to get used to the taste, so they then offer baby drinks or juice instead, which are generally sweet and go down much more easily. Of course, once a child gets used to flavoured drinks, she's unlikely to be happy with plain water.

Why is water important?

A good fluid intake is essential because dehydration can lead to headaches, poor concentration and constipation. Sugary drinks (fruit juice, juice drinks or squash) are a major cause of tooth decay. They also contribute to a child's energy intake. So if your little one drinks lots of juice between meals she may be too full to eat at mealtimes, or she may be consuming too many calories in total, and therefore become overweight.

Drinks with artificial sweeteners may seem a healthier compromize, but children still develop a taste for over-sweet drinks, and there is some concern about the safety of artificial sweeteners for children. So the bottom line is: water really is the best non-milk drink.

Action plan

O Offer water and don't give babies any other drinks (except milk) until they are happily drinking it.

O If you are concerned about dehydration, give them food that is more watery, such as juicy fruits, and make baby meals runnier by adding a little water.

O Babies may object to plastic cups, so try giving them water on a spoon or from an open cup at first. Then, when they are used to drinking water, go back to the lidded cup.

O Let a toddler choose a new cup or drinks bottle in the shops. Then use this ONLY for water.

O If the water level seems to stay the same no matter how much she sucks, check she is able to use the cup: some non-spill lids require industrial suction to get anything out.

O For toddlers hooked on juice drinks, gradually dilute them more, and then offer plain water.

O Keep giving water. The more you do, the more likely they are to drink it. If they leave half a cup, it's not a big waste!

O Make an agreement with older children about when they will have water and when they can have other drinks. For example, they could have water at lunchtime and between meals, but diluted fruit juice with supper. If they never drink water, having a cup with one meal would be a start.

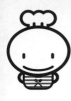

Vetoing vegetables

This is probably the most common food problem among children. Although it is recommended that everyone should eat five portions of fruit and vegetables a day, the average child eats only half this amount.

Babies tend to enjoy a variety of vegetables, but when they become toddlers these are often the first foods that are pushed aside. Parents who insist a child eats vegetables before he gets any pudding only exacerbate the problem: it reinforces the idea that vegetables are horrible, but pudding is enjoyable. It would be interesting to see what would happen if you encouraged your child to eat pudding first and only then allowed him to have a beautiful broccoli tree.

Why are vegetables important?

Vegetables contain essential vitamins and minerals, including antioxidants, as well as fibre and phytonutrients, which provide a range of health benefits. Eating lots of vegetables boosts the immune system and reduces the risk of heart disease and certain cancers.

Eating fruit can partly compensate for a lack of vegetables in a diet, but it doesn't contain all the healthy substances found in vegetables. High intakes of vegetables in childhood are associated with a lower risk of stroke in later life, but high intakes of fruit don't offer the same protection. Also, vegetables generally have fewer calories than fruit, so they are important in energy balance and weight management.

Action plan

O Hide vegetables in foods children like. This will make it possible to increase their intake without too much resistance. Start with small amounts and gradually increase them.

O Keep serving up new vegetables and don't anticipate rejection every time. A child who hates peas and carrots may surprise you by liking spinach, broad beans or red cabbage. So provide a wider variety more often and keep them coming.

O Serve raw vegetables such as carrots, peppers and cucumber with a dip as a starter.

O Provide small portions of vegetables. Serving just three slices of carrot is less likely to cause an argument and it will stop you worrying about waste. It is also less daunting for a vegetable hater.

O Don't offer children other foods as a reward for eating vegetables, or threaten to withhold pudding.

O Let them see you eating and enjoying vegetables.

O Teach them why different vegetables are important (see Chapter 4).

O Offer them a choice, for example: 'Do you want carrots or broccoli?'

O Make food more fun and get the children involved in choosing vegetables when in the supermarket, arranging food into a picture or colouring in a Gimme 5 hand (see page 202).

O Counter cries of 'I hate vegetables!' by reminding your child of any they do like – even if it's only baked beans and carrot cake.

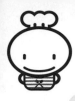

Ten places to hide vegetables

1   Mashed potato or cheesy mash, such as parsnip, swede.

2   Pasta sauce (use a blender to disguise peppers, broccoli, and so on, if necessary). Lasagne is especially good for this.

3   Pizza topping, for instance mushrooms, finely chopped peppers, peas, sliced tomato.

4   Cake, such as carrot, courgette.

5   Risotto. Instead of serving chicken, rice and vegetables separately, cook them together.

6   Soup, for example, tomato and lentil, leek and potato.

7   Roast vegetables, such as parsnips, carrots, peppers, along with roast potatoes or potato wedges.

8   Veggie burgers.

9   Baked beans, for example, grated carrot or courgette.

10 Sandwiches, wraps and pitta pockets, for example, tomato, watercress.

No fruit

Refusing to eat fruit is less common than hating vegetables, probably because fruits are sweeter. However, some children seem to dislike the texture of fruit, or they may tolerate bananas and nothing else. They may have enjoyed puréed fruits as a baby, but when it comes to crunching on a raw apple or chewing an orange segment, it doesn't have the same appeal.

Why is fruit important?

Fruits offer many of the same health benefits as vegetables: they are rich in antioxidant vitamins, minerals and phytochemicals, which have anticancer properties. In addition, children who eat plenty of fruit are less likely to suffer from asthma. Children who won't eat fruit tend to get less vitamin C and may have insufficient amounts of other essential nutrients, too.

Action plan

O Offer your baby pieces of fresh fruit as finger food as soon as she can manage them (six to nine months), for example, peeled pear, melon, peach.

O Try lots of different fruit, then you're bound to find something she likes. Fresh, frozen, tinned and dried fruit are all good.

O Give her fruit as a snack, such as sliced apple and pear, raisins, dried apricots.

O Hide fruit wherever possible:

⊙ Smoothies, for example, blend banana, strawberries and orange juice

⊙ Add stewed or mashed fruit to yoghurt

⊙ Cakes, such as apple, banana, dried fruit

⊙ Freeze fruit purée into cubes and defrost for sauce on ice-cream

⊙ Make ice-lollies with fruit juice or fruit purée

O Have fun with fruit by chopping it up and making funny faces or boat pictures.

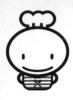

- Serve a wide variety of fruit regularly and present it in different ways:
    - ⦿ Kebabs with grapes, strawberries and pineapple cubes
    - ⦿ Half a kiwi fruit in an eggcup with a teaspoon
    - ⦿ Thick slices of banana, with a fork to spear them
    - ⦿ Half a peeled kiwi speared on a baby fork as a lollipop
- Talk about the benefits of different coloured fruits and try some of the activities described in Chapter 9.

Bland foods – yummy!

The problem of liking only bland foods seems to develop most commonly around the age of two (see Chapter 1). In extreme cases, this can mean that a child turns down all colourful food such as green vegetables and red or orange fruit and eats only white, beige or yellow products, such as bread, pasta, chips, cereal and cheese. Children may also eat chicken but refuse salmon or red meat. This seems like an incredibly boring diet to parents, but as long as your child is still eating some fruit and vegetables he is unlikely to suffer nutritionally.

Often this kind of fad occurs when children become increasingly exposed to the wider world – perhaps starting nursery or just becoming more aware of their surroundings. Some experts believe children may find it comforting to have a bland and predictable diet when their environment is expanding and they are experiencing new stimuli in other areas of life.

However, this fussy eating may also develop simply because these are the kinds of foods the child has been given to eat most often, because they require little or no preparation and are often thought of as acceptable children's food.

Action plan

o Stop worrying. Your child is very unlikely to become malnourished on these foods and will probably grow out of it.

o Start by increasing the range of accepted foods: for example, offer slightly different kinds of bread, a variety of pasta shapes and even coloured pasta twists. This should stop him becoming too rigid in his likes and encourage him slowly to expand his dietary repertoire.

o Try giving fruit and vegetables that appear the least threatening, such as mashed or roast parsnips, slices of peeled yellow pear or apple purée.

o Try some of the steps suggested for children who won't eat vegetables and fruit (pages 114–18).

Allergies and food intolerance

We all know that the incidence of food allergies is rising in children, and if your child is a sufferer it can be a worry. It is currently estimated that 14 per cent of under-fives and 10 per cent of five- to ten-year-olds have some form of food allergy, according to parents' reports. However, the figure for allergies that have been officially diagnosed by a doctor is lower, at around 5 per cent for all children under 10. Cases of food intolerance are thought to be more common, but there are no official figures to confirm this.

The most common foods to cause allergies in children are milk, eggs, nuts, fish, soya and wheat. Most children with allergies to milk and eggs grow out of them, but this is less likely to happen with nuts, fish and shellfish. Allergies can produce a range of symptoms, including behavioural problems such as hyperactivity, as well as rashes, wheezing, stomach upsets and allergic rhinitus (itchy eyes and a runny nose). It is not understood why, but behavioural problems are more commonly reported among boys and eczema is more prevalent in girls. The most serious form of allergic reaction is anaphylactic shock, which is very rare but can be fatal. It involves symptoms occurring in different parts of the body at the same time, including rashes, swelling of the lips and throat and breathing difficulties.

It can be difficult to recognize an allergy or intolerance in your child. Generally if she gets the same reaction every time she eats a certain food and the reaction begins very soon after consumption, you can be fairly sure it is an allergy. Less commonly, symptoms may not appear for a few hours after a child has eaten a food she is allergic to. Allergic reactions are usually fairly immediate because they involve the immune system, which reacts as soon as the body comes in contact with a particular food by releasing chemicals to fight it. The immune system mistakenly recognizes proteins in the food as being harmful, and it is the chemicals your body produces in response to this that result in the adverse symptoms experienced.

Occasionally children experience symptoms such as bloating or an upset stomach after having a particular food, which is due to food intolerance rather than an allergy. If this is the case, the reaction doesn't involve an immune response and probably isn't so immediate. It is thought that psychological factors play a role in some cases of food intolerance but others have a well-established biological cause, including lactose intolerance and coeliac disease. In these conditions, children don't produce the enzymes needed to metabolize milk and wheat products, respectively.

Action plan

O Don't try to diagnose an allergy or intolerance yourself. If you suspect a problem, see your doctor who can then refer your child for tests at a hospital. Many health-food shops and private clinics offer tests, but these are often expensive and generally unreliable. Without a proper diagnosis your child may be avoiding foods unnecessarily.

O As there is no cure, the only way to prevent a reaction is for your child to avoid the food she is sensitive to.

O If your child is allergic or intolerant to a whole food group, such as dairy foods, ask your child's doctor to refer you to a dietician so that you can check she is getting all the nutrients she needs from other foods.

o Learn to read food labels so you can recognize any alternative names that may be used to describe the food your child has to avoid (see Resources at the end of the book).

o Tell your child and anyone who cares for her – including hosts of children's parties – exactly what your child can and can't eat. Also tell them what to do if she does accidentally eat something she shouldn't, including how to use an adrenaline pen (Epipen) if she has one.

A vegetarian diet

It may be your choice or theirs that your child has a vegetarian diet. Babies sometimes decide they don't like meat, probably because of the texture, but this is often temporary and passes as more teeth appear. Older children may want to stop eating meat because of concerns for animal welfare or limited global resources, or because they believe a vegetarian diet is healthier. Vegetarian friends may influence them or they might simply dislike the taste of meat. If they give you a legitimate reason for becoming vegetarian, you should respect their choice. While a diet without fruit or vegetables will be less healthy than a mixed one, a diet without meat needn't be.

If your child is particularly worried about her body weight, it is possible that she is giving up meat to reduce her calorie intake. Some research suggests that young girls in particular may adopt a vegetarian diet to cut down the amount they eat without generating resistance. Becoming a vegetarian is generally more acceptable than announcing you're no longer going to eat breakfast cereal or bread, for example.

A vegetarian diet can be healthier than one including meat. Vegetarians have been found to have lower blood cholesterol and lower rates of hypertension (raised blood pressure), heart disease, type-2 diabetes, and colon and prostate cancer. However, it's not clear whether these benefits are due to diet or lifestyle factors linked to vegetarianism – such as not smoking, doing more exercise or drinking less alcohol.

A vegetarian diet does need careful planning to ensure it's healthy. Cutting out meat and eating chips and cheese instead, with very little fruit and vegetables, is likely to lead to anaemia and a feeling of being lethargic and run-down. Vegetarian convenience foods, such as sausages and burgers, are not always a healthy option as they can be high in fat and salt.

Parents sometimes complain that their child wants to be a vegetarian, but doesn't like beans or lentils, or any vegetables come to that. This obviously makes it difficult to get all the nutrients she needs from the few foods she is eating. It is generally easier to plan a healthy diet for a child who is a lacto-ovo-vegetarian (one who eats eggs and milk) than a vegan (who excludes all foods of animal origin – such as meat, chicken, fish, eggs, milk and honey).

Vegetarian nutrition

When planning a meat-free diet you need to be particularly vigilant to ensure an adequate intake of the following nutrients:

Nutrients	Vegetarian sources
Protein	milk and dairy products, eggs, beans and lentils, soya products such as tofu
Iron	breakfast cereals with added iron, beans and lentils, dried fruit such as apricots
Zinc	cheese, leafy green vegetables, nuts and seeds, tofu
Calcium	milk, dairy products such as cheese and yoghurt, soya products with added calcium
Vitamin B_{12}	milk, dairy products, eggs, soya products with added vitamin B_{12} , yeast extract, such as marmite
Omega 3 fatty acids	flaxseed and rapeseed; many foods now have omega 3 fats added

Tips

Protein needs are better met by having different protein foods at the same time, such as beans on toast or lentils with rice.

Have some vitamin C at the same time (such as orange juice, broccoli, kiwi fruit) to increase iron absorption.

Make sure not all meals have wholegrain cereals, as the phyate they contain reduces zinc and iron absorption.

Calcium shouldn't be deficient in a vegetarian diet, but vegans should have soya milk or puddings with added calcium.

Vitamin B_{12} isn't found naturally in vegetarian foods, so read food labels to make sure you include foods with it added in.

If a food claims to contain omega 3, look carefully to see just how much it has and that it is 'long-chain' since this is the most beneficial.

Action plan

O For a baby who dislikes meat because of the texture, you could try shepherd's pie or other dishes with minced meat or chicken. Also give meat alternatives such as beans and lentils.

O If your child is underweight ensure that she has plenty of energy-dense foods like avocados and crushed nuts and seeds. A vegan diet in particular can be very bulky for young children, so they feel full before they've eaten enough calories and nutrients.

O Think about the foods they will eat and how they can get a balanced diet from them.

O Discuss with your child what she will eat but don't argue with her about it. Would she be happy to eat free-range meat? Does she want to eat chicken? Perhaps she would like to eat meat occasionally, depending on her reasons for wanting to become a vegetarian. What about fish? Eggs? Or milk, cheese and yoghurt?

O Talk about how your child is going to ensure she gets all the nutrients she needs within the framework of a vegetarian diet. Take into account practical considerations. For example, are you going to cook a separate meal for her every day? Perhaps the whole family could eat a vegetarian meal or some fish (if she will eat it) a couple of times a week. It might even improve everyone's diet. You could freeze extra portions of vegetarian meals or make batches of dishes such as vegetable and lentil sauce or chickpea curry for other days.

O Eat together as a family whenever possible. Often at least part of a family meal will be vegetarian-friendly. Your child could eat the same potatoes and vegetables as everyone else, but have something else instead of meat. Or have a different sauce when you cook pasta. This way she is more likely to eat well and you will still get all the other benefits of eating together (see pages 31–4).

O If you're concerned that your child isn't growing properly or could have anaemia or other health problems, talk to your doctor or health visitor.

O Learn more about vegetarianism by visiting the website for the Vegetarian Society or Vegan Society (see Resources at the end of the book).

Don't forget

O Relax. Fussy eating usually passes and children are very unlikely to become malnourished during this time – think of 'Jam Boy'!

O Never force a child to eat anything.

O Refusing certain foods can be a way of asserting independence and some control, so making a fuss can be counterproductive.

O Children's tastes can change frequently and unexpectedly, so try to be patient.

O Teach your children about nutrition and how they can look after their body.

O Get them involved in choosing and preparing food so they have some control.

O Keep at it. Children need to be given different foods many times before they accept them.

O Write a list of small realistic goals, and keep trying to reach the next one.

Refusing to eat

It can be very worrying when a child refuses to eat. Food is so intrinsically linked with our sense of nurturing, that having a little one who turns it down can make you doubt your parenting skills. But try to remember he is rejecting only the food, and his behaviour doesn't mean you are a bad parent. Your task is to provide him with healthy food: it is up to him whether or not he eats it. That said, there might be particular factors behind his behaviour which you can identify and resolve. If nothing else, you should certainly be able to reduce the stress that you, and probably he, feels at mealtimes.

Take some comfort in the knowledge that, while severely restricted diets are associated with poor growth, most difficult eaters do not appear to be at risk nutritionally. If children eat when they are hungry and stop when they are full, most will grow to their expected size.

So what's the problem?

Many parents worry that their child seems to survive on nothing but air. In reality, though, she must be getting some food. Even for children who refuse proper meals, the little bits they do eat and the snacks in between add up. Keep a food diary to see what your child consumes over a few days: a close look at this could put your mind at rest, or help you to identify particular problems (see page 136). It's also worth getting your child weighed and checking growth charts to see if she is genuinely underweight.

It's not uncommon for parents to overestimate the amount of food their children need. A study of nearly 500 five-year-olds in Finland found that 30 per cent were thought to be poor eaters by their parents. These 'poor eaters' did have a lower absolute calorie intake, but this was because they were smaller, and so needed less. When calorie intakes were adjusted for body weight, there was no difference between the 'poor eaters' and the rest. The only difference between the diets of the poor and good eaters was that the poor eaters received fewer calories from main meals and more from snacks. (It should also be noted that these children had been smaller at birth, so their lower weight was not as a result of poor eating habits.)

If after analysing your child's growth it is revealed that she is underweight, it is a good idea to look into ways to increase her dietary intake (see Children who live on air on page 140). However, if she is a poor eater but her weight is OK, this can be addressed another way (see Grazers on page 142).

Why won't my child eat?

Parents of toddlers often worry that their child seems to have gone off food, but in actual fact a smaller appetite is normal at this stage, as children's growth slows down in the second year of life. Also, toddlers experience an increasing sense of independence, and a refusal to eat is a common expression of this newfound autonomy. Knowing what to expect from your child at different stages of his development may help you to understand his behaviour better (see Chapter 1).

It can be difficult to know whether your child is refusing food because he doesn't like it, or because he isn't hungry, or because of a behavioural issue. One way to determine this is to ask yourself whether your child behaves the same way when he's in a different setting or when you're not around. If he eats better at Granny's house or at nursery, then it might be that he is refusing to eat at home because he enjoys seeing your reaction, or at least finds it interesting.

There are many reasons why children may not eat much at mealtimes. We often look for complex explanations for a child's behaviour and miss the more obvious things. It may simply be that he wants to run around and play; or he might not have a comfortable seat (if his feet are dangling and he can't reach the table properly, he's more likely to want to get down). Perhaps dinner is offered to him too late and he's too tired to sit down to a civilized meal; or perhaps he is scared of making a mess when he eats or using his cutlery wrongly and being told off for it. It might just be that he finds mealtimes boring, particularly if he eats alone or is not included in the conversation. Children love to hear stories about when you were a child, but they are less interested in hearing you discuss moving your mortgage. The opposite may also be true – there might be too much stimulation at mealtimes: if the TV is on or other activities are taking place in the room, this could be distracting him from the task at hand.

If your child refuses to eat, you may come to dread mealtimes and the coaxing, the arguments and the tears that follow. In this situation it can be difficult to create the kind of atmosphere that is most conducive to eating, but it could be what makes all the difference. While food should be the main focus of a meal, a little light conversation could help reduce the pressure your child might be feeling.

Common pitfalls for anxious parents

If a child doesn't eat at mealtimes, parents are often tempted to give unhealthy snacks instead, thinking a biscuit is better than nothing. But this action will result in a poor nutrient intake and can perpetuate the problem.

Children are surprisingly good at regulating their energy intake and keeping it at a similar level from day to day. This means that if they consume lots of calories from biscuits, or even milk, they will take less from foods such as potatoes and meat, thereby missing out on the essential nutrients these contain. Also, if snack foods are available, they may decide not to eat lunch because they prefer biscuits. If your child is regularly skipping certain foods such as vegetables or meat, you will need to use specific techniques to ensure she doesn't miss out on key nutrients (see Chapter 5).

Parents will often cajole a child to try foods she dislikes or to have 'just one more spoonful'; and in the past, some children

were made to sit at the table until they had cleared their plate. While these strategies are well intended, they can turn mealtimes into a power struggle. They also tell children to eat for external reasons rather than in response to internal body cues, which teaches them that even if they feel full, uncomfortable or ill, they should eat. Small children are good at recognising when they have eaten enough and when to stop eating, and this is something that you don't want them to unlearn.

Another issue can be that a parent simply lets the child leave the table if she's not eating. This gives the child the message that there is a choice – you can eat or you can play. Given the option, many children, especially toddlers, will choose to play. By making it clear that this option isn't available and if they don't want to eat they should still sit and chat at the table, they might stay and even eat a little more.

Children should be encouraged to eat when they're hungry and to stop when they're full. They shouldn't be eating to please you, or be refusing food just to annoy you.

Keep tabs on growth

You can find out how well your child is growing, compared to others his age, by plotting his height and weight on growth charts. If your child has a 'personal child health record' (the red book you were given by the health visitor when your baby was born), these charts are at the back. If you don't have this red book, visit www.healthforallchildren.co.uk. Your health visitor will usually weigh and measure babies and pre-schoolers for you; otherwise it is easy to do it yourself.

If your child's weight is below average but still correct for his height, then there shouldn't be any cause for concern. For example, if his height is around the 25th percentile, it is reasonable for his weight to be around the 25th percentile too (that is, he is taller and heavier than a quarter of his age group). Across the population, some children will inevitably be shorter and lighter than others. However, if your child is on the 75th percentile for height, but, say, the 9th percentile for weight, there may be an eating issue you need to investigate. Of course, height and weight graphs rarely follow smooth lines, and sudden growth spurts and periods of stability are normal, but if your child's weight drops several percentile lines – for instance from the 75th to the 25th – you should seek advice.

It is important to remember that growth is not the only indicator of children's well-being. You should also ask yourself: Are they generally healthy? Do they rarely get ill? Have they got plenty of energy? Are they happy? If the answer to all these questions is 'yes', the fact that they are underweight may not be quite as worrying as you think.

However, if all these questions make you think your child isn't growing properly, talk to your health visitor or GP. Growth can be affected by a hormonal imbalance or a problem with nutrient absorption. Your doctor should be able to investigate these further, or rule them out and put your mind at ease.

Keeping a food diary

In order to get a proper idea of your child's diet, write down everything she eats for at least four days. If you feel you are not seeing any patterns after this time, carry on for up to seven days. Below is an example of what your food diary should include.

Tips for keeping the diary:

- Write down every single thing that was eaten, even a few raisins – little bits all add up.
- Include all drinks, apart from sips of water.
- Write things down as they are eaten or drunk, or you won't get a complete record. It doesn't have to be neat; it's just for you. Don't try to remember later or keep scraps of paper.

Time	Location	What was given
7am	kitchen and bedroom	cup of milk
7.30am	kitchen table	bowl of Shreddies
8.30am	pushchair	½ banana
10am	Tom's house	1 chocolate digestive orange squash

○ Include anything that might be useful, such as whom they ate with.

When you look at the food diary, try to identify problems which you can then tackle. It may help to ask yourself some questions when you look at it. For example:

○ Has she had snacks too close to mealtimes?

○ Could too much milk or juice have made her full?

○ Did she regularly miss out on any particular foods, such as fruit and vegetables?

○ Were lots of unhealthy snacks eaten?

○ Did she eat more when she ate alone? With the family? With other children? In front of the TV? In the pushchair?

○ Could she have been too tired to eat?

What they had	Anything else
cup of milk, plus extra ½ cup	cried for more milk while I was getting things ready
2 spoonfuls	big argument, rushing out of the house
½ banana	sister's banana
1 biscuit ½ cup	same as Tom - they ate together

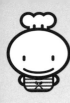
Dos and don'ts for handling food refusal

Do

O Structure eating: provide three meals a day with two snacks in between at regular times.

O Get your child to sit at the table during mealtimes, even if she doesn't eat.

O Make sure meals aren't too late and are not given when he's overtired.

O Check her seat is comfortable and at the right height for the table.

O Keep portions small: big plates of food can look over-whelming. If he eats it all, he can ask for more.

O Relax and take a step back – pressurized mealtimes are not conducive to eating.

O Make mealtimes enjoyable, but avoid too many distrac-tions. Eat together whenever possible.

O Allow your child to stop eating when she says she's had enough.

O Make every bite count. (That means giving them healthy meals and healthy snacks.)

O Encourage more involvement in preparing food or plan-ning meals.

Don't

O Nag your child to eat throughout the meal or make any threats.

O Force a child to eat anything, or insist on 'just one more spoonful'. You can decide on the foods, but he should be allowed to decide how much he eats.

O Hurry a slow eater; if she's eating happily, then give her the time she needs.

O Insist a small child uses cutlery properly and doesn't make any mess.

O Make a child sit at the table until *you* think he's eaten enough. If he's just sitting and not eating then keep him there for a while, but be aware that 15 to 20 minutes is about the limit, then you should let him get down.

O Look disappointed or give the impression that a child has let you down by not eating.

O Give unhealthy snacks between meals, especially close to mealtimes.

O Give too much milk or juice to drink between meals.

O Keep offering her food or asking if she's hungry between meals.

One step back...

Don't be discouraged by setbacks – there will inevitably be times when your child goes off his food again. Try not to worry; perhaps he feels off-colour or doesn't fancy what you've cooked today. The best way to cope with his food rejection is not to over-react, but to re-read the list of dos and don'ts (pages 138–9) to make sure you're handling things in the best way. This setback doesn't mean your new approach hasn't worked, so don't go back to bribery or putting undue pressure on him: you'll just undo your good work. Instead, try to relax and keep at it.

Children who live on air

Some children simply have a small appetite and little interest in food. This can be particularly difficult for parents to understand if they see food as one of the great pleasures in life.

Young children are sometimes said to be 'failing to thrive' if they are not growing and putting on weight as quickly as expected. The phrase has no widely accepted definition, but it is often used for those whose weight is below the 5th percentile. Another term sometimes used by the media is 'muesli malnutrition'. This refers to middle-class children who are underweight because they are fed a low-fat, high-fibre diet under the mistaken belief that it is good for them. There is no evidence to suggest this is a widespread problem, but it does highlight the need for young children to be offered foods such as meat and cheese in their diet, and not too many bulky ones such as muesli and wholemeal pasta. If you are unsure about the types of foods that are appropriate for your child's age, see Chapter 4.

When a child is underweight it's very tempting to give her anything that she'll eat. However, chocolate and other treats will provide only the calories and not the vitamins and minerals she needs for healthy development. So, instead, look for foods which are energy-dense, but also dense in nutrients.

Action plan

o Take the pressure off eating and make mealtimes enjoyable occasions when you all chat and spend time together.

o Limit the amount of high-fibre foods in your children's diet, such as brown rice and muesli. These are bulky and can make them feel full before they get enough nutrients and calories.

o Avoid low-calorie foods such as diet drinks, fat-free yoghurts, or snacks such as rice cakes.

o When you cook, don't skimp on the vegetable oil, and maybe add a bit of olive oil into pasta towards the end of cooking.

o Offer your children high-density foods, such as cheese, avocado, full-fat yoghurt, peanut butter (or other nut or seed butters) or dried fruit.

o Go for nutritious drinks such as fruit smoothies, milkshakes or yoghurt drinks.

- Make sure snacks and drinks, other than water, are given a long time before meals.
- Try eating in different places, such as having a picnic lunch in the park.
- Consider giving them multi-vitamin and mineral supplements, but make sure they are specifically made for children.
- See your doctor or health visitor if you are worried.

Grazers
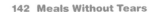

Some children appear not to eat much but somehow they are not underweight, so they must be getting the calories they need from somewhere. Although they may be reluctant to sit down to a proper meal and they might say they're not hungry, the little bits they do eat soon add up. This is another instance where keeping a food diary can be very revealing. When you count up a few sweets in the pushchair, a couple of biscuits at playgroup and another on the way home, it might suddenly explain why they have a poor appetite at lunchtime.

Grazing is most common with toddlers and pre-school children. They are simply too busy to stop what they are doing to sit down and eat a proper meal, and when they do sit down at the table they are easily distracted. These young children also have a small appetite, which means they can't eat a lot at one sitting and therefore need snacks between meals. Another problem may be that mealtimes don't coincide with periods when they are hungry: at lunchtime they might only eat a little because they're ready for a nap, so then they are ravenous by mid-afternoon, which in turn means that when supper comes along, they're not hungry. In this case, a re-think on meal scheduling might be all that is needed.

You might have read that people who eat little and often are healthier and less likely to be overweight than those who enjoy large meals. However, the danger for children who don't eat proper meals is that the snacks they have consist of unhealthy foods such as biscuits, sweets and crisps. If this is the case, they're then likely to eat fewer vegetables and protein foods, such as meat, fish and eggs, which they need for healthy development.

Children who drink lots of milk also tend to eat less at meals, and those who have more milk than they need are likely to have lower iron levels – particularly when milk is drunk at the expense of meat, fish and foods which enhance iron absorption, such as fruit.

For toddlers who like to graze, think of snacks as 'mini-meals' and include some protein foods along with fruit and vegetables. As children approach school age, they are able to eat more at one time and should become less reliant on snacking. If you encourage a pattern of having three proper meals a day, they are more likely to eat well in the long term.

What a child eats is more important than when they eat.

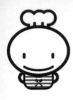

Action plan

O Make sure your children see you sitting down and eating proper meals, rather than just snacking throughout the day. If you eat together, it will also help to keep them focused.

O Reconsider the eating environment. Do they have comfy chairs? Is cutlery a problem? Are there too many distractions, such as toys or the TV?

O For toddlers, make snacks 'mini-meals' and give them a slice of cold pizza, vegetable sticks and houmous, cubes of cheese and an oatcake or fresh or dried fruit.

O If your child has hungry times of day which don't coincide with meals, would a schedule re-think be possible?

O For children of school age, try keeping snacks healthy but not too big, such as a piece of fruit or a rice cake, and see if this improves their appetite at mealtimes.

O Make sure they aren't getting all the energy they need from milk or juice, which will leave them too full to eat proper meals.

Good eaters who suddenly refuse to eat

Adults tend to eat about the same amount of food every day, which is largely due to habit. We are less responsive to appetite than our children; they are more likely to eat, or not eat, in response to hunger and satiety cues (feeling full), which means they can seem to have nothing one day and then be ravenous and ask for seconds and thirds the next. It may seem unsettling, but it is not worth worrying about. A balanced diet, particularly for children, doesn't work on a daily basis. If you keep a food diary, you are likely to see that over about a week their intake will look reasonable.

You should really have cause for concern only if your child's lack of appetite continues for more than a few days; in this case it could be that he is ill or teething, but if so there should be other signs in addition to a drop-off in appetite. If you are worried, talk to your GP or health visitor.

Action plan

O Even if your child is not eating, stick to your regular meal and snack routine and at these times just offer him small amounts of food.

O Don't worry about a decline in appetite, unless there are other signs of illness or he doesn't eat for several days.

O When your child is not eating, try to remember that this has happened before and he made up for it when his appetite returned.

O Allow him to choose the amount he wants to eat: whether this is a lot or a little. But don't allow him to choose between healthy food and junk foods.

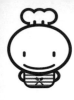

Breakfast dodgers

You will often hear people say that breakfast is the most important meal of the day, yet it is the one that is skipped by people of all ages more often than any other. Some children just can't seem to face eating in the morning, even if they have had nothing for 12 hours.

This situation can be testing when you're in a hurry to get everyone ready and out of the house, or just to get on with the day. However, by allowing them to skip breakfast you are running the risk that they will be hungry by mid-morning and will be asking for unhealthy snacks instead.

Creating a breakfast routine is not just about avoiding bad snacking habits. Children who don't eat breakfast have been found to have lower intakes of fibre and certain micronutrients, particularly vitamins A and C, riboflavin, calcium, zinc and iron. This is because most breakfast cereals are fortified with iron and a range of vitamins, and because children are more likely to have fruit juice, milk and high-fibre foods at breakfast than later in the day. So if your child misses breakfast but is hungry later, it makes sense to give her cereal mid-morning, if possible. (She can even have breakfast cereal as a mid-afternoon snack if she'll eat it.)

As well as having a better vitamin and mineral intake, children who eat breakfast are less likely to be overweight. This may be because they generally eat fewer high-fat snacks than breakfast skippers, or because they tend to be more physically active.

Good foods for breakfast

O Different breakfast cereals or porridge.

O Sliced banana, raisins or yoghurt, and so on, added to cereals to make them more interesting.

O A boiled or scrambled egg with toast (preferably wholemeal).

O Baked beans on toast and a glass of orange juice.

O Yoghurt and fruit.

O Cheese on toast.

O A fruit smoothie or fruit and yoghurt blended together.

Breakfast on the go:

O A banana.

O A sandwich (preferably made with wholemeal bread), with a filling of cream cheese, cheese, ham, peanut butter, banana or jam (if nothing else will do).

O Oatcakes with cream cheese or marmalade.

O A drink, such as milk, 100-per-cent fruit juice, a smoothie or a yoghurt drink.

Research has shown that eating breakfast has a profound effect on performance at school; those children who do so score higher in memory and academic tests. One American study also found that giving breakfast to children who usually skipped it led to fewer cases of depression and hyperactivity.

Cereal bars might seem the obvious solution for children who won't eat a proper breakfast. Some claim to contain milk and wholegrain cereal. This sounds great, but in fact most contain about 40 per cent sugar – which is more than a chocolate digestive biscuit. The idea of giving breakfast skippers something they can eat on the way to school, is, however, a good one, but try to choose something healthier.

Action plan

○ Make sure toddlers aren't having a big drink of milk immediately before breakfast. If possible, give it to them earlier or have breakfast later. Perhaps you could provide less milk in the morning and they could then have more later in the day, if they need it.

○ Include some complex carbohydrate and protein foods if possible, such as wholegrain cereal and milk or wholemeal toast and egg.

○ Try some different breakfast ideas.

○ Get children involved in thinking of something healthy that they might like to try.

○ If toddlers won't eat breakfast, have something healthy ready for them to eat mid-morning.

○ Get older children to take something they would like to eat on the way to school.

When hunger hits at bedtime

Children who eat very little during the day sometimes complain that they are 'starving' at bedtime. It may be that their need for food has finally caught up with them, but don't underestimate how clever your child can be. If he knows you are concerned about him not eating enough, then food is the ideal tool to delay bedtime. By going back to the kitchen and preparing more food you may rest easier for today, but you won't solve the problem. He will probably not eat dinner again tomorrow, and you could be creating a new problem at bedtime.

You may feel like a terrible parent if your child goes to sleep hungry, but there is a big difference between sending him to bed without any dinner, and giving him dinner but allowing them to choose whether or not to eat it. If he decides not to eat and you respect this, he will learn from the experience.

At the same time children can also learn, with your support, that most decisions don't have terrible consequences and can be rectified. They may go to bed a bit hungry, but they can have a big breakfast in the morning and have another chance to eat tomorrow evening. Resist the temptation to say, 'I told you so;' instead, be positive. Tomorrow, it will be up to them again to choose whether or not to eat dinner.

Action plan

● If they don't eat dinner, warn them that this is their last chance to have any food until tomorrow. They have the choice of eating now or waiting until breakfast.

● If they choose not to eat, let them live with the consequences – that is, going to bed hungry.

● Be supportive and show that you respect their decision.

● If there is a long time between the evening meal and bed – for example dinner at 5pm and bed at 8pm – serve the dinner later.

Watching their weight

As children get older they become increasingly aware of the pressure to be thin and may refuse food in an attempt to control their weight. This is particularly true of girls, but increasingly boys are starting to show concern over their image and a desire for thinness. From a very young age, children are given the idea that 'thin = good'. They are bombarded with this message by the media, the internet and their peers: images of waif-thin supermodels and singers inevitably affect a girl's perception of body weight, and about how fat or thin she is compared to the norm. Likewise, well-toned footballers and singers sporting six-packs can affect a boy's self-image.

Children may hear you and other adults, or indeed their friends, talking about dieting, so it's important to tell them that, in reality, diets don't usually work. Even people who lose lots of weight generally put it back on again. Try to impress upon them, too, that dieting and being underweight can also result in serious health problems.

This fascination with dieting and being thin is not exclusive to teenagers; children as young as seven have been found to develop eating disorders. So if your child complains about her fat tummy, don't dismiss it. That said, severe conditions such as anorexia nervosa and bulimia nervosa are rare, although the key features of these disorders – such as an obsession with slimness and body dissatisfaction – are all too common.

Try to encourage your child to have a good self-image and realistic, healthy expectations of how she should and can look. You can promote a positive self-image by giving her the right sort of compliments – those that don't just focus on her physical appearance, thereby shifting her own focus on herself, too. For example, by all means mention how nice your child's hair looks, but also remember to say how she makes you laugh, how good she is at drawing or how you love her smile.

Children who are trying to lose weight sometimes decide to skip breakfast or stop eating certain foods, such as dairy products. These sorts of diets mean they will miss out on crucial nutrients such as calcium and iron, so talk to them about eating a balanced diet. Remind them about healthy eating and why they need different foods and repeat the message that they should eat when hungry and stop when full.

Encourage your children not to develop too rigid an attitude to food: they can still eat their favourite foods, as long as it is in moderation as part of a balanced diet. Even eating salad all the time isn't a balanced or healthy diet. If your child is overweight, be supportive of her desire to slim down, but try to teach her that losing weight through starvation is not a good idea (see page 185).

Action plan

○ Give your child regular meals, including breakfast, which are well balanced.

○ If she isn't very physically active, encourage her to walk and exercise more.

○ Be a good role model yourself. If you are concerned about your own weight, consider how your worries might affect your child (see Chapter 3).

○ Promote a healthy and balanced attitude to food: it's not bad to eat chocolate sometimes.

○ Don't fight her desire to take more control over what she eats. Instead, give her choices and encourage a sense of responsibility.

○ If she is aware of super-thin celebrities, talk about them and encourage an interest in healthy-weight role models. Make sure you know who she's interested in, as comments about role models from your own childhood or teens aren't going to get the message over!

○ If you are worried that your child is losing weight, see your doctor or contact one of the organisations which deal with eating disorders (see Resources at the end of the book).

Don't forget

O Try to relax and remember that a healthy child who eats when he's hungry and stops when he's full will grow to his full potential.

O Never force a child to eat.

O Keep a food diary to see how much your child is really eating. Use it to identify particular problems and to see how things could be improved.

O Look at your child's growth charts to see if she is really underweight.

O Don't dread mealtimes: they should be an enjoyable time to be together, even if your child chooses not to eat.

O If you are worried, talk to your health visitor or GP.

Trouble at the table

Children will be children, but if mealtimes look more like a chimpanzee's tea party than an episode of *The Waltons*, it's time to take action.

With some youngsters, the trouble starts as soon as you say, 'Dinner's ready,' and it can be a battle just to get them to the table. With others, so much food is plastered on their hair, clothes and everywhere else within a 1-metre radius that you wonder if any has actually reached their mouth at all. Whether they are constantly leaving the table, starting food fights or burping competitions, or indulging in any other misbehaviour, all in all it doesn't make for a pleasant dining experience.

Manners, please!

As they get older children generally begin to eat a wider range of foods and become more willing to try new things. However, parents are also more likely to experience an increase in bothersome behaviour and general bad manners at mealtimes.

Part of the problem is that when they are at the table children have a captive audience for their antics. They know you want them to stay there and eat, and they also know that therefore you're less likely to punish them then than at other times. If there are other distractions at mealtimes, such as the TV or toys, these can add to the general mayhem. So the key to avoiding this chaos is to make eating a more focused activity: if children are sitting at a table with other people, they are more likely to be better behaved.

If you've been on holiday to France, Spain or elsewhere in Europe, you may have watched in awe as local children sat politely in a restaurant, eating adult food and enjoying a family conversation. So there's proof that it can be done. Children are quite capable of eating a meal in a civilised manner if they are brought up to enjoy good food and conversation. Eating together regularly as a family is crucial if you want to teach your children good table manners. (Among other benefits, it can also help to encourage children to eat a better diet – see page 32 for more on this.)

By teaching children from an early age how to behave during meals, you will also feel more confident about taking them to eat at other people's houses and at restaurants. In addition, if they find themselves in different social situations in later life they won't feel intimidated, but will be able to enjoy such occasions. It does take effort but it can be done, and the dos and don'ts on the next page will help.

Messy eating and food throwing

When babies and toddlers eat they inevitably make a mess. Whether they are using a spoon or their hands, they will sometimes miss their mouth and end up with food on their face, their clothes and the floor. You may think they're doing it to annoy you but, to begin with at least, they're just learning and experimenting; finding out which foods are crumbly or squishy and what happens when they push food off the side of the highchair.

In such a scene you might be tempted to rush in with a cloth and wipe up the mess immediately – but don't. Doing this can give your child the idea that messy food is bad, and it might put him off eating. Mess is just something that you have to

Do

O Sit down with your child at a table while he eats. If possible, try to eat the same meal, or just have a drink or a snack with him.

O Make sure your child is seated at a comfortable chair which is the right height for the table.

O Give children sufficient warning when it's nearly time to eat so they can finish up what they are doing, or get them involved in preparing for the meal: for example, helping with the cooking or laying the table.

O Praise good behaviour. You could even try a reward chart with stickers for staying in the chair until the end of the meal, using cutlery nicely, or being polite, etc. (Always draw attention to their positive rather than negative behaviour. For example, talk about 'sitting nicely', rather than 'not putting feet on the table'.)

O Create a pleasant dining experience for all by staying calm and displaying good manners that they will, hopefully, copy.

accept and try to minimize, if you can. Don't be tempted to take over and feed your toddler to spare the mess; the only way he is going to learn to feed himself is by having a go.

Sometimes this behaviour can turn into something of a game, with a toddler intentionally throwing or dropping food because they enjoy seeing your reaction – whether it's

Don't

O Have the television on while your child is eating.

O Have toys, or anything else that could cause a distraction, on the table. Babies sometimes need something in their highchair to keep them happy, but older children don't. If this doesn't work, perhaps favourite toys could sit somewhere else and have their meal while your child eats his.

O Pay attention to bad behaviour, unless it's really getting out of hand.

O Nag children about eating up, finishing their vegetables, learning their spellings, or anything else during the meal. Instead have other topics ready to discuss, such as an upcoming party or outing, or even how you're dying to hear about what happened in *Bob the Builder* today.

laughter or exasperation. The best thing to do in this situation is to try not to react at all, however tempted you are. If you find more food is being thrown, dropped or spread than is actually being eaten, it's probably a sign that he's had enough. If this is the case, end the meal and let him get down.

Action plan

- Minimize mess by:
  - Covering the floor with a splash mat or newspaper.
  - Rolling your child's sleeves up above the elbow.
  - Using a large bib with a pocket for catching bits.
  - Keeping portions small. (He can have seconds later if he is still hungry.)
- Try to ignore any mess until the end of the meal.
- Provide distraction from intentional food throwing by sitting with your child while he eats.
- Encourage self-feeding: if necessary put a spoon in each hand and give him part of the meal as finger food: for example, carrots on the side, rather than mashed or chopped up with the rest of the meal.
- Choose foods that are easier for self-feeding. Meals such as shepherd's pie, fisherman's pie or Weetabix stick to the spoon quite easily. A baby who likes to eat with his fingers will find pasta bows easier to pick up than spaghetti, and slices of pear easier than puréed pear.
- If your child has had enough, get him down from the table.

Spitting out food

We all know the saying about taking a horse to water. Well, the same goes for a baby: you can give her food, you can even put it in her mouth, but you can't make her eat it.

You might find that your baby spits out any food you give her, or that she simply opens her mouth and lets it fall out. This can often happen when babies start weaning simply because they're not used to having solids and they aren't quite sure what to do with them. As they get used to this new food, though (and this is usually within a week, if not days), they should get the hang of moving it to the back of their mouth and swallowing it.

Babies who have gone beyond this initial stage of weaning may also spit out food. If this is the case and your child's expression is telling you she's not enjoying it, take the hint and stop feeding. For someone who can't talk, this is the only way she can get her message across. She either doesn't like the food, or you're going too quickly and she needs a rest, or she's had enough. If you keep on trying and offering her food, you're only going to make yourself frustrated and her upset.

When an older baby or toddler spits something out, she may be doing it for attention or to show you that she doesn't want you feeding her. If she is eating with other children and she can't join in by talking, it can be her way of getting noticed. If you react by making a fuss, or if other children start laughing, it will inevitably egg her on. The best solution is to give only positive attention. Encouraging self-feeding may also help.

Action plan

- If you're feeding your baby and she's spitting out the food, stop and think why she is doing it.

- Ignore the food spitting if you think it might be for attention and take steps to minimize the mess.

- Try to give positive attention and provide some distraction – you can chat to a baby even if she can't talk back.

- Encourage self-feeding by giving her a spoon and foods that can be eaten easily.

- If your child is obviously spitting out food just for fun and no tactic is stopping her, warn her, then take the food away.

Refusing to come to the table

You know your child is hungry, but as soon as you call, 'Dinner is ready,' he reacts as if you'd just announced that Christmas is cancelled. This may then be followed by claims that he's not hungry, and by the time he reaches the table he's in such a bad mood that when he sees the meal he'll say he hates it, whatever it is.

This kind of behaviour often has little to do with the meal itself, but more a reluctance to leave whatever activity the child was doing before. Children often get very engrossed in what they're doing – whether it's watching TV, building a tower or playing a game – and some need extra help in changing activities.

You may find that it's not just mealtimes that cause this problem; getting washed or preparing to leave the house might prompt a similar outburst. This behaviour can be exhausting, but there are steps you can take to help him to make the transition from playing to the table much easier.

First, the child needs some warning that he will need to go to the table soon – imagine how you would feel if you had almost finished cooking a meal, or you were in the middle of watching a cup final, and someone said you had to stop immediately. You probably wouldn't react too well, but an advance warning might have made things easier.

Giving your child an activity to do in between playing and eating can also help, even if it's just washing his hands. Then, if your child is still angry about having to stop playing, he can vent his fury at the sink, rather than at the table. Asking your child to help get the meal together might also help: if he enjoys laying the table or calling everyone else for dinner, he will be more able to see the meal as a shared activity, rather than as a chore. If your child usually plays in another room but eats in the kitchen, getting him to move from one room to the other might be easier if he does something at the kitchen table, such as drawing, for a while before his meal.

Another problem may be that children see meals as a time for arguments and scolding, which inevitably puts them off coming to the table. This scenario might have evolved because of the stress of getting your child there, but when he does reach the table, you need to try to forget this and

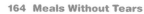

instead endeavour to create a calm atmosphere with pleasant conversation. Focusing on the mealtime itself, as well as the pre-meal preparation, should help your child to see it as a more enjoyable experience, which should also ease the transition to the table.

Action plan

○ Give your child at least two warnings that it's nearly time to eat, perhaps ten and five minutes beforehand. He might not have much concept of how long this is, but he should get a sense that it is soon.

○ If your child finds it easier to understand, tell him he'll be eating at the end of the TV programme he's watching, or after he's finished the picture he's drawing.

○ Make sure you're not serving dinner when he's in the middle of watching his favourite TV programme.

○ If children need help in ending their play, perhaps you could suggest that a doll goes for a nap or that the cars go and park in the garage. This also shows that you respect what they have been doing.

○ Get your child involved in preparing for the meal by washing hands, helping to make some part of the meal, or laying the table.

○ Try to make mealtimes relaxed and enjoyable.

Attempting the great escape

With some children, getting them to the table is only the start of your problems: keeping them there long enough to eat a meal is the real challenge. They may sit for a few minutes, eat a small amount and then say they've had enough, or they might simply stop eating altogether and decide to get down. It's at this point that parents will either attempt to get them to stay and eat more, which might result in a full-blown tantrum, or allow them to get down, which tells them their behaviour is acceptable.

Again, it's worth having a think about the environment in which your child is eating, and if this has any influence on her behaviour. If your child is a toddler and has progressed from a highchair to a booster seat or normal chair, it may be that the move was made too early. Your child might be thinking that since she's now physically able to leave the table, she can therefore get down when she pleases. As a rough guideline, most children aren't ready to change chairs until at least two, because before then they are unlikely to understand why they should stay put.

Another factor may be that small children have a limited attention span and might want to leave the table because they find mealtimes boring and would rather be doing something else. However, even toddlers should be able to stay at the table for at least fifteen minutes. In order to help them do this, try to make mealtimes about more than simply eating. If a child gets down after just a few minutes, the chances are that her initial hunger has been satisfied but she won't really have eaten enough to fill her up. So she'll be asking for snacks before long. While you shouldn't insist on a child actually eating, you should be able to get her to stay at the table and chat for a reasonable amount of time. If she does begin to slide away under the table or start to get agitated, then distraction is the best way of averting a tantrum.

If that fails and a tantrum ensues, you could try ignoring it: although that can be difficult when you are sitting at a table, especially if you're trying to eat and talk to someone else as well. Also, if your child is having a really good tantrum, then it's unlikely that she will be able to stay on her chair, so it might be necessary to remove her for a while until she calms down. Don't allow her to play in this calming down time, though, or you'll just be rewarding her bad behaviour. Once she's had a few minutes of calm, bring her back to the table and try to start a pleasant conversation again.

Action plan

O Consider whether you have moved a toddler from her highchair too soon. If so, get it out again or buy a booster seat with a good seat belt.

O Get your child involved in the meal by getting her to help you with its preparation.

O Include your child in the conversation so that she doesn't get bored and want to leave the table.

○ Make the mealtime atmosphere as pleasant as possible.

○ As far as behaviour goes, try to keep the focus on staying at the table, not on eating the meal.

○ If your child has a full-blown tantrum, calmly remove her from the table to quieten down for a few minutes, then bring her back and immediately try to resume friendly chitchat.

Mealtime mayhem

When your child is young, you might think there could be few things worse than him spitting out food or spreading it over the highchair or his hair, but just wait until your child eats with other children more often – particularly those with older siblings.

This is the time when you could find yourself treated to burping and food-cramming competitions, food throwing or flicking, plate licking, proud displays of half-chewed food, feet on the table and jokes about a variety of bodily functions followed by uncontrollable giggling. You might smile at the thought and even recall your own childhood antics, but when it happens at every meal it can be very tiring. If you're thinking how fortunate you are that you don't have to contend with all of these at the moment, don't rest on your laurels; now is the time to encourage good table manners so that, with any luck, you will never have to face this.

Good table manners don't involve children sitting rigidly at the table with their elbows by their sides, or being able to select the correct fork when faced with a regiment of cutlery;

they just mean knowing how to eat and talk with other people in a civilized way. Children should be encouraged to sit normally – not slouching sideways over the table or standing beside it – and they should be aware that they shouldn't talk with a mouthful of food.

As children get older they can gradually be taught more about what sort of behaviour is acceptable at the table. While a small child can't be expected to sit in his chair for a long time, an older one can be told that it's polite to wait until everyone has finished before he gets down. Likewise, an older child should know how to use cutlery properly and, if he has to burp (which he will probably insist he does), do it quietly and say 'excuse me' afterwards. (If he is older, he should also be perfectly capable of understanding that it's not polite to burp loudly and then roar with laughter afterwards!)

Taming bad behaviour and encouraging good manners should go hand in hand. As with other issues, children are more likely to behave well and appreciate their food if they have a part in its preparation and if they enjoy the social aspects of eating together. And remember, it's perfectly possible to share a joke and have fun during a meal without bad manners.

Action plan

○ Try to ignore bad table manners and instead praise any good behaviour.

○ Keep the conversation flowing. Use the time during a meal to get to know your children better by encouraging them to share their ideas and views. If this doesn't come naturally to you, it might help to think up a few topics in advance.

○ Have a 'posh dinner' occasionally. Put on some music, have a candle on the table and let everyone get dressed up. If your child helps to choose the menu or prepare the food, he will get a sense of pride in and responsibility for the meal, which should help him behave when it comes to eating it. He could also make a table decoration or pick some flowers for the table, and when you are all sat down you could talk to him especially politely, or even pretend to be a waitress. This isn't something that you need to do regularly, but it can help break the cycle of mealtime mayhem. Then, whenever things start slipping out of control again, you can organise another occasion in order to get him back on the right track.

○ Try a reward chart and give your child stickers or stars for specific types of good behaviour, such as sitting nicely for the whole meal or only making polite noises (that is, not burping loudly) during it.

○ An appropriate reward for good table manners might be that you take your child out to eat in a restaurant.

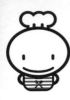

Eating out with children – never again!

Taking children to eat at a restaurant can be a real test of their table manners, and you might even feel that your parenting skills are also on trial if you start receiving disapproving looks from fellow diners. If your child is screaming for ice-cream, having a tantrum or running around wildly and knocking over glasses, you're bound to feel embarrassed; but ask yourself if she is really behaving any differently from how she would at home, or is it simply more noticeable in a restaurant?

Many parents hope their child will rise to the occasion and behave well in public, but this isn't always the case. Sitting down to a meal and having a pleasant conversation is a skill, like any other, that children need to learn – and if they don't practise it at home, how will they know what to do when in public? When you're out with friends it's important to remember to include the children in the conversation, otherwise they may well get bored and misbehave to get your attention.

You might think the key to getting good behaviour from your child is to go to a restaurant that provides balloons, and crayons, and perhaps even a ball pit. While these can be fun sometimes, the food isn't usually that tasty or healthy and, more importantly, your child won't be learning how to enjoy a proper meal out. Also, in a few years she'll be too old for such places and you will be left with the same problem.

Eating out as a family or with friends can be great fun, and an opportunity to enjoy good food and lively conversation, so it really is worth cultivating the skills your child needs in order for her, and you, to get pleasure from it.

Action plan

O Practise eating out at home by having a 'posh dinner' or playing restaurants.

O Prepare children for the occasion in advance by telling them how you are expecting them to behave.

O Choose a child-friendly restaurant: you don't need to go to a fast-food burger chain, but perhaps try a local Italian restaurant where children are welcome and it's not too formal.

O If you have a toddler or a very small child, have something that she can play with at the table or nibble on, like a rice cake. She will probably expect to eat as soon as she gets to the table and may find it hard to wait.

O Don't put your child in a highchair as soon as you get there, or she'll be itching to get out by the time the meal arrives. Instead, let her sit on your lap or move around a bit, if there's room.

O Go out at a time when your child would normally eat. If she is over-hungry or very tired, the dining experience is likely to be less than ideal.

O Bear in mind that ordering a starter will stretch out the meal, which might not be a good idea. Small children in particular may last better if you go straight to the main course. If you're eating with other people who want starters, ask for your child's main meal to come at the same time as these.

- Include children in the conversation.

- Be prepared to leave if your child misbehaves. Warn her that if she chooses to behave badly, it's not fair on other people and that you will have to take her out of the restaurant. Then, if necessary, you need to carry through on this threat.

Don't forget

O Babies and toddlers make a mess when they eat. This is how they learn to feed themselves and they can easily be cleaned up after the meal.

O Bad behaviour at the table may be a cry for attention, so try ignoring it and instead encourage good behaviour with distraction, conversation and praise.

O Children may object to being called to the table for meals because they are engrossed in other activities. An advance warning and strategies to ease the transition from play to table can help.

O While you shouldn't insist your child eats, it is reasonable to expect even a small child to sit at the table for at least 15 minutes.

O If you promote an interest in food and encourage conversation at the table, children will be more likely to want to stay and behave well.

O Good behaviour and table manners have to be learned, and therefore taught.

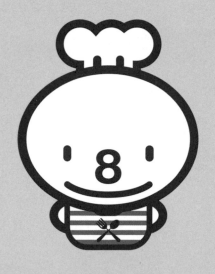

Problems of excess
– overeating and
weight problems

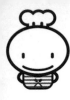
Children who enjoy their food are often affectionately described as having hollow legs and, likewise, a hearty appetite is seen as a sign of good health. But if your little one is regularly consuming more food and calories than he needs, he will inevitably become overweight and thereby increase his risk of ill health. Eating problems that develop early in life can persist into adulthood, so it is vital to address them as soon as they arise. However for children, even more than for adults, it is important to think about healthy eating in general, not just in relation to their weight or size.

Problems of excess can take different forms: some children seem to eat all the time or constantly complain of hunger, others may polish off meals without appearing to stop for breath, and some might continually demand unhealthy junk food. One or all of these behaviours may sound familiar, whether your child is overweight or not.

An increase in appetite is a normal response to a growth spurt or lots of physical activity, but when calorie intake is greater than energy needs, problems can start. It is also worth investigating if this is happening because your child is turning to food for the wrong reasons. Even an average-weight child can develop an unhealthy relationship with food and, while this may not pose an immediate risk to his health, it could increase his chances of becoming overweight or obese in the future.

For a growing number of children the effects of eating too much, combined with a lack of physical activity, are evident. More than a quarter of two- to ten-year-olds in England are overweight and more than 10 per cent are obese. In Scotland about one in five children is classified as obese – a higher proportion than even in America. Obesity is often perceived to be a problem for older children who spend too much time playing computer games and eating fast food. However, it is now increasingly affecting children of primary school age, and even pre-schoolers.

The issues covered in this chapter differ from others in this book because they cause fewer obvious everyday problems for parents (compared with behaviour such as refusing to come to the table or spitting out food). However, carrying excess weight does pose both immediate and long-term risks to a child's health and well-being. Some parents might have their own problems with overeating, excess weight and poor body image, and this can make addressing their child's issues all the more difficult. So think about your own weight issues, and how they might affect the way you feed your child, before you decide your little one really does have a weight problem and how you should go about tackling it (see Chapter 3).

Is your child overweight?

Some parents worry unduly that their toddler's round tummy is an early sign of obesity, while others explain away their child's excess weight as puppy fat. It has been found that, although mothers generally know when they themselves are overweight, they are not always so good at identifying weight problems in their children. In a study of overweight two- to five-year-olds, it was found that 80 per cent of the mothers did not recognize their child was overweight. Part of the problem may be that in the first few months, or even years, of a child's life, the focus is on getting her weight up, and so it might not occur to parents that it is increasing too rapidly.

The percentile charts in your child's 'personal child health record' (the red book you were given by the health visitor when your baby was born) are helpful as a first indicator of whether your child may be overweight. If the percentile for weight is

So when is a child obese?

It is more difficult to assess whether a child is overweight than an adult, but your doctor will probably use BMI (body mass index) charts as a guide. (These aren't in your child's red book, but can be viewed on www.healthforallchildren. co.uk.) If an adult has a BMI greater than 30, he is described as obese, but a similar cut-off point cannot be set for children. This is because their proportions, and the relationship between their height and weight, change as they grow. Generally, a child over two years is defined as being obese if her BMI is above the 98th percentile for her age – which means her BMI is higher than 98 per cent of her peers. If a child's weight falls between the 91st and 98th percentiles, she will simply be described as overweight.

much higher than that for her height, talk to your heath visitor or doctor about whether your child has a problem. Likewise, if your child's weight jumps up several percentiles – say, from the 50th to the 91st percentile line – it could also indicate that something is wrong and might need addressing.

If you find out that your child is overweight or obese, you need to take action – don't just hope she will grow out of it.

So my child is overweight – does it matter?

The simple answer is, yes, it does. Being overweight or obese in childhood has serious implications for health and can also put children at risk of social and emotional problems, such as bullying and low self-esteem.

The dangers of obesity in children are similar to those facing adults, including raised blood pressure, increased blood cholesterol and elevated insulin levels. A study of overweight five- to ten-year-olds found that 60 per cent of them displayed at least one of these three signs, putting them at an increased risk of developing cardiovascular disease. Another problem emerging among very overweight children is early-onset type-2 diabetes. This can result in serious complications, including the loss of limbs and blindness in severe cases. Childhood obesity is also associated with orthopaedic problems, fungal skin infections, liver problems and psychological illnesses.

If your child is overweight but not actually obese, or if he is very young, it can be easy to dismiss these risks. However, elevated cholesterol levels have been found even in moderately overweight children, and the initial stages of atheroscelosis have been shown to occur in children as young as three years. This condition shows itself when fatty deposits start to develop in the lining of their arteries, which could later lead to a heart attack or stroke.

In addition, being overweight or obese as a child increases the chances of growing into an overweight or obese adult. This has been shown in several large population studies that have demonstrated a quite obvious tracking of weight problems from childhood into adulthood.

If your child does have a weight problem it is not inevitable that it will continue into adulthood, but, equally, it is unwise to assume that it will simply disappear with time. As has already been mentioned, parents of tweenies will often excuse their child's weight gain as 'puppy fat' and believe it's perfectly normal for children to be a bit chubby before puberty starts and they get a growth spurt. For some children this is genuinely what happens, but it's not necessarily the case across the board.

Although it's not unusual for some weight gain to occur in these early years, it can also be a warning sign of things to come. A study of girls in America found that those who were overweight at nine years old were nearly 15 times more likely to be overweight in early adulthood.

Why do children overeat?

You might be concerned that your child sometimes overeats, even if she is not actually overweight, but there's no need to be concerned if once in a while your child eats too much at a friend's party. However, if she seems to eat very fast or consume very large amounts, and it isn't because of a growth spurt or lots of physical activity, warning bells should start to sound.

Sometimes children, like adults, eat for the wrong reasons – they may be bored, upset or tired. Giving children food as a reward, especially junk food or sweets, can lead to them associating these foods with the good feeling they have when they've achieved something. Likewise, giving sweets to children to soothe them after they have hurt themselves can encourage them to turn to food for comfort later. Similarly, using food to keep children quiet, or to stop them complaining of boredom on a car journey, can give them the message that snacking is a leisure activity.

Most parents do these things occasionally without any obvious ill effects. However, regularly using sweets or other foods in these ways can result in children forming unhealthy associations with food. So, while it's fine to give children sweets occasionally, be careful as to how you do it and bear in mind any negative messages you might inadvertently be sending.

The upshot is that it is important that you help your children to develop a healthy relationship with food by encouraging them to eat when they are hungry and learn to distinguish hunger from other emotions. Remind them that hunger is a feeling in their tummy, not usually in their mouth or anywhere else. If your child is asking for food because she is bored, remember that boredom can be cured by far more satisfying activities than eating.

While helping your child to recognize the emotions she is feeling, get her to understand that everyone has nasty or uncomfortable feelings sometimes – such as anger or jealousy – and while she can't stop these feelings arising completely, she can acknowledge them and discover alternative outlets for these emotions.

Finding extra time in a hectic lifestyle to talk though problems with children can be difficult, but it can make a big difference to them.

Sometimes small children overeat because they don't have enough control themselves at mealtimes. Toddlers and older children who are still spoon-fed can eat too much, particularly if they are very compliant, which can lead to them eating more than they really want or need, and ultimately to excess weight gain. It's important to stop feeding a child when she indicates she's had enough – even if it means throwing away carefully prepared meals. So as soon as children are able to start feeding themselves, they should be encouraged to do so for their own good.

Older children might overeat because they aren't aware of how different foods affect their body. Messages about food and weight are everywhere, and many of them are misleading.

So unless you ensure your child understands the basics of nutrition, she's unlikely to know what she should really be eating. Also, if she usually eats in front of the TV, she may be so absorbed in what she is watching that she doesn't notice what she is eating, or register when she is feeling full. By improving your child's understanding of food and by getting her to enjoy healthy meals in a pleasant environment (without distractions such as the television), she will become more in touch with the food she is eating.

Ready access to highly palatable but unhealthy junk food is another problem sent to try parents who want their child to eat healthily. Chapter 4 looks at how best to handle the issue of junk food with children, but esentially you need to make sure they don't have unlimited access to foods such as biscuits, crisps and sweets, and instead are provided with plenty of healthy alternatives for snacking on.

Tackling your child's problem with excess is not easy, and it may require difficult changes to many aspects of her, and your, lifestyle. This is where your influence as a role model is enormous. However, to prevent your little one becoming part of the much-publicized 'child obesity epidemic', you need to rise to the challenge.

Do

○ Talk to a health professional to establish whether your child actually is overweight or obese.

○ Get toddlers to feed themselves.

○ Encourage your child really to think about whether she is hungry and to distinguish hunger from other feelings.

○ Ensure your child has regular nutritious meals, including breakfast, and that fruit and other healthy foods are available to her as snacks.

○ Be a good role model and eat with your child whenever possible.

○ Serve meals in a pleasant sociable environment without distractions.

○ Teach your child about healthy eating and get her involved (see Chapter 9).

○ Ensure your family enjoys plenty of physical activity together.

Don't

○ Ignore a weight problem and simply hope your child will grow out of it.

○ Use food as a reward or to comfort a child who is hurt, upset or bored.

○ Allow children to eat unhealthy snacks while they sit and watch television.

○ Keep a readily accessible store of sweets, crisps and biscuits in the house.

Helping an overweight or obese child

Admitting that your child has a weight problem and recognizing the increasing health risks he faces can be difficult. If you or other members of the family are overweight, you might put your child's problem down to genetics; but don't use that as an excuse to avoid trying to help him. While genetics do have a role to play in some cases of obesity, upbringing is critical.

Researchers have identified several lifestyle factors that increase the likelihood of children becoming overweight. One study, involving 8000 children of primary school age in America, came up with some interesting results. It found that the risk of becoming overweight increased for every additional hour of television viewed per week, and that the risk decreased each time in a week that the child ate with his family. While you can't do anything about your child's genetic make-up, it should be reassuring to know there are things you can do to help him in other ways. So, as a first step, why not reduce screen time to no more than two hours a day and try to eat as a family as often as possible? Just these two simple changes to your lifestyle could make a real difference to your child's weight.

Even if a child has an underlying predisposition to put on weight, the bottom line is that children become overweight because they consume more calories than they use. Therefore, if you want to tackle your child's excess weight you need to address both sides of the equation: he needs to eat more healthily and he must become more active.

However, weight-loss programmes aimed at adults are not suitable for children and rapid or uncontrolled weight loss is rarely recommended for young children. Instead, your doctor may think it is appropriate for your child to slow down his rate of weight gain or simply to try to maintain his current weight. Then, as he grows taller, he will reach an appropriate weight for his height. Remember, children have specific energy and nutrient requirements for growth and development, so it's important to listen to what your child's doctor recommends.

Whenever you talk to your child about his weight, sensitivity is vital. He needs to know he is loved and supported and that you are not criticizing him, otherwise he might become defensive about the issue. If you also have a weight problem, admit it; and whether or not anyone else in the family has a problem, you all need to work together. Trying to impose rigid rules on one child, but not on his siblings, can have negative effects, so it is vital that healthy eating guidelines apply to everyone in the household, while still ensuring that each child has a diet appropriate for his age (see Chapter 4). A better diet and some extra physical activity aren't going to do anyone any harm.

Getting started

Keep a food diary (see page 136) to make it easier to identify where the extra calories in your child's diet are coming from. When you're putting a new, healthy-eating programme into action, start by making small changes and gradually introduce more modifications. For example, instead of providing biscuits after school, offer some fruit. Or, instead of having chips five days a week, serve them just twice. Once your child has changed one bad habit, he can start on the next. If you set short-term goals, it will help keep everyone focused and maintain motivation.

Rather than talking about 'dieting' with an overweight child, it's better to focus on 'healthy eating'. There is no quick-fix solution, and the road to healthy eating is long: your child needs to adopt eating habits that he can follow for the rest of his life. The ultimate goal is that your child will be able to manage his own eating and weight in later life.

Getting your child involved in making a plan and setting goals is particularly important for weight problems (see page

Little steps

The more changes you can make over time, the better, but even small alterations can have a significant effect. A study of seven- to eleven-year-olds in Dorset found that by cutting down on fizzy drinks by a third, they were able to halt the rise in obesity over a year. In contrast, a control group of children experienced a 7.5 per cent increase in the rate of obesity over the same period. The improvement in health was made by just reducing their consumption of fizzy drinks, and without making any other changes to diet or physical activity.

217). Self-motivation is essential because if a child feels you are imposing rigid rules, he may rebel and overeat when he gets the chance. Likewise, if you ban certain foods, he might just become obsessed with them.

A child should be told it is okay to eat when he's hungry, but to think first about whether he might really be thirsty, or perhaps just bored. Then if he does want something to eat, think about what he eats rather than how much: so he should be offered plenty of fruit, vegetables and high-fibre foods which will sate his appetite better than processed foods and snacks.

To help your child change their eating habits for the better, try to encourage an attitude of moderation and flexibility. Whatever your child's favourite food, he should be able to have it sometimes. So if he eats some chocolate he shouldn't feel bad or guilty, but know that everything is OK in moderation. Many adults take the view that once you've eaten something 'bad', you've blown any healthy eating for the day, and therefore you might as well just pig out and start being good again tomorrow. This is an unhealthy attitude which is characteristic of yoyo dieters: you need to help your child adopt a more balanced approach to eating and treats.

In order to help your child control his weight you will have to accept the role of baddie sometimes. This can be easier if you agree parameters with your child beforehand, but it's still up to you to stick to them. So if you agree that he can have one chocolate bar a week and he decides to eat it on

Monday morning, you should respect his decision and allow him, and you, to live with the consequences. If he is very upset about not having chocolate for the rest of the week, be sympathetic, but don't give in – he will learn by the experience. If the week is very tough you could allow him to have two chocolate bars the following week, but make the rule in advance and stick to it.

Again, family environment is hugely important in managing weight problems. The more often children see you eating and enjoying healthy meals and snacks, the more normal healthy eating will seem. Likewise, they should see you taking exercise and walking, not sitting in front of the box and complaining about feeling tired. Studies have found that strategies to reduce sedentary behaviour and increase physical activity are particularly useful in treating childhood obesity, especially when parents are included.

We know that following weight loss adults often regain the pounds they've managed to shed. However, the good news for children is that by using healthy eating and physical activity to control their weight they are more likely to be successful in the long term than adults.

Action plan

- Make small and gradual changes.
- Focus on what your child eats, not just the amount.
- Encourage him to have more of the following foods and drinks:

- ⊙ Plenty of water
- ⊙ Wholegrain cereals and bread
- ⊙ Fruit and vegetables – aim for at least five a day of a variety of these in place of foods higher in fat and calories (give him something fun like a pineapple if he's feeling deprived)
- ⊙ Low-fat dairy products (only for over-twos)
- ⊙ Lean meat, skinless chicken and fish (without any batter or other coating)

○ Encourage him to have fewer foods and drinks which are high in calories, fat and sugar:

- ⊙ Carbonated drinks, squash and even fruit juice (it still contains sugar, so it will increase calorie intake)
- ⊙ Fried food
- ⊙ Crisps, chocolate and sweets
- ⊙ Processed foods, such as ready-meals and sausages
- ⊙ Pizza and other dishes with lots of full-fat cheese

○ Pay attention to portion sizes, particularly with snack foods and when you're eating out.

○ Get your child moving (see page 211).

○ Make healthy eating fun by planning meals and cooking together. Focus on cooking low-fat foods with plenty of vegetables or salad.

○ Get the whole family involved.

Finishing a meal without taking a breath

Sometimes children become very focused on eating and they don't appear to notice what is going on around them, or hardly pause for breath. They may even look surprised when their plate is empty and immediately ask for more, or panic slightly. You might notice this happens more often when they are very hungry, or if they're eating a food they especially like.

Behaviour like this can occur at any age, but most often it develops in pre-schoolers. Children who have trouble moving from one activity to another can be especially susceptible, and although the ability to focus and not be easily distracted is valuable for studying, this isn't so when it comes to eating. If children become so engrossed in the sensations of eating, they won't know what to do when they are finished. They might have been very hungry before they started, but by bolting their food there isn't time to notice when they are full. So these speed eaters need to pause, maybe have a drink and a chat, and then think about whether they are still hungry.

This kind of behaviour must be addressed as early as possible because when they have access to unlimited amounts of food in the future, it might develop into binging.

Of course, getting a hungry child to pause between mouthfuls can be easier said than done. After about 10 seconds, she'll probably tell you she's had a break and is ready for seconds, but she needs to learn that it takes time for her body to realize she has had enough – at least five or ten minutes. It may help if she is allowed to start a new activity; if chatting isn't enough of a distraction, perhaps she could draw for a while. Then, once she's got into something else, she may decide she's not really hungry after all, and thus learn a valuable lesson.

However, if after the agreed five or ten minutes' wait she is still asking for more food, let her have it – even if you think she's had enough. To allow your child the space to change her behaviour, she needs to know that she can eat if she's hungry, otherwise you risk losing her trust and undermining her confidence in making her own decisions. You want to help her to understand her body's needs, so that she will be able to eat a sensible amount when you're not there taking control.

Action plan

O Give children regular meals and snacks to make sure they don't reach a point where they are completely starving.

O Try to slow down the rate at which they eat by chatting about things they're interested in, or perhaps asking them to pass you something across the table.

O Don't cut up their entire meal, as this makes it easier to eat quickly.

O Make sure portions aren't too big, then they could have seconds (after a rest).

O Encourage them to taste the food properly by asking a question about it while they eat, such as, 'Do the carrots taste crunchy, or are they soft?;' 'When you eat the fish with the potato, does it still taste the same?' Or anything else that springs to mind that will get them thinking about the food they are eating.

o If they want more, reassure them they can have more if they still feel hungry in a little while.

o Teach them that it takes time for the 'hungry' or 'full' message to travel from their tummy to their head, and they need to listen for it carefully.

o Away from the table, talk about eating until you feel like you've had enough, and not eating until you feel uncomfortable or sick.

Always hungry, and always after a snack...

Some children always seem to be hungry, and you might wonder if they do in fact have hollow legs. They've just finished dinner, but they're already reaching for the biscuit tin and saying they need a snack. Sound familiar?

Very occasionally, constant hunger can be due to a rare genetic disorder called Prader Willi syndrome, which is characterized by an insatiable appetite. But for the vast majority of children, a closer look at their eating habits may reveal something simpler. It may be that when they say, 'I'm hungry,' what they really mean is, 'I want some sweets,' or 'I want a biscuit.' However, if only bananas or other healthy snacks are on offer, they might suddenly decide they're not really as hungry as they'd thought.

If you teach your child about nutrition (see Chapter 4), he will learn that different foods do different things for his body, so you can tell him sweets taste nice but they don't make you healthy, so it's better to eat something else – such as a piece of fruit or toast – if he's hungry. Then if he wants a few sweets afterwards, he could have some.

If a child is hungry, it's not fair to deny him food; if you do, it's likely to result in fights or secret eating. However, if you have doubts about whether he really is hungry, check that he's not just thirsty, bored, or is in need of some emotional comfort. It's difficult to establish whether this is the case every time, but there may be clues; such as if he is wandering around aimlessly then saying he's hungry, or if he is grumpy or quiet except when he's eating.

Don't threaten your child with 'you'll get fat!' when he asks for more food, as this may increase negative feelings and a sense that his eating is out of control. Instead, help him to think about whether he is really feeling hunger in his tummy, or something else. Don't do this every time he complains of hunger, but when you have the time and it seems appropriate.

Reinforce the message that he knows better than you if he is really hungry and if he is, you will, of course, always allow him to have something to eat. This shows you respect his ability to know what is best for his body and also helps him to become more confident that he can make good decisions.

Action plan

O Help your child to distinguish hunger from other feelings (see page 181).

O Reinforce the message that only he knows if he's really hungry, not you.

O Have healthy snacks ready when you know he's going to be hungry, such as:

   ⊙ Vegetable soup

   ⊙ Sticks of raw carrot, cucumber, celery and pepper

   ⊙ Fruit

   ⊙ Rice cakes

O Avoid comments like, 'I'm sure you've had enough now' or 'You can't still be hungry,' as these will undermine the child's confidence in knowing his own body.

Don't forget

O Speak to a health professional if you think your child is overweight or obese.

O If your child has a weight problem, don't just hope he'll grow out of it.

O Help your child to distinguish hunger from feeling thirsty, bored or upset.

O Just because you or other family members have a weight problem, it doesn't mean you can't help your child.

O To achieve healthier eating, make dietary changes small and gradual.

O Think about healthy eating rather than dieting, and increase intakes of water, high-fibre foods and fruit and vegetables.

O Remember that physical activity is just as important as diet when it comes to managing weight – so get moving.

O Parents are fundamental to treating children's weight issues, so if your child has a problem, don't feel there's nothing you can do or leave it up to someone else to resolve.

The road to a more enjoyable family life

By the time you reach this chapter, I hope that you will have gained lots of useful tips to try out. Don't worry if there is too much to remember – just take it one step at a time. Getting children to eat healthily and happily isn't something you can achieve overnight and then forget about: it's an ongoing process. As your little one grows older, her relationship with food will change and different issues will arise: you may find that the toddler who worried you by eating nothing can't get enough food when she becomes a tweenie.

Whatever stage your child is at, and even if you have no specific problems, it's worth bearing in mind the five dos and don'ts from Chapter 2. I've re-capped them here as they are the key to helping your little one have a balanced diet and to establish a healthy relationship with food. If you follow these guidelines, mealtimes should become much less stressful for both you and your child.

Remember: start by making small and gradual improvements to the way you and your family eat. Any more than this and you risk overwhelming both yourself and your child.

Do

1 Lead by example.
2 Offer a healthy balance of foods.
3 Teach your child about food and nutrition.
4 Eat together.
5 Relax and trust your child.

Don't

1 Make a child eat anything.

2 Label your child.

3 Be too rigid with your child or yourself.

4 Give food as a reward or for comfort.

5 Allow too much TV.

Who's worried now?

If you find it hard to stick to these dos and don'ts and you are constantly trying to control what your child eats or are worrying about her uneaten meals, you might benefit from thinking more carefully about your own relationship with food (see Chapter 3). The role of food in your upbringing and your current feelings about weight and how much you eat will inevitably affect the way you feed your family. Sometimes a child's apparent 'problem' may have more to do with the parent's own anxieties. By looking more closely at these issues, you should be able to separate them from your child's eating habits and in doing so, you will be better able to help her form a healthy relationship with food.

To enable your little one to develop a balanced attitude to eating, it's important to create a positive food culture at home where healthy eating is the norm but treats are not demonized. Chapter 4 sets out the basics of nutrition and includes a table

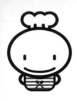

of 'nutrition facts for children' to help you teach your child more about what he's eating.

Your child is more likely to take the advice on board if he gets involved in choosing or preparing food, so on pages 202–7 are 10 healthy eating activities which should give you some inspiration as to how to get him involved. You can adapt them or use them as a starting point to devise new ways to encourage a positive relationship with food.

The key to success with these activities is to keep things relaxed and maintain a balanced approach. For example, bake cakes together as well as making fruit salad or vegetable kebabs, because you don't want to teach him that cakes or other treats are 'bad', as this can promote an obsession with healthy eating.

All these activities also have the added bonus of allowing you to spend some quality time with your child, which is an important thing for your relationship with him and will help him to feel a valued member of the family.

However busy you are, you should be able to make some improvement to your child's eating habits. This is about his future health, after all, and what could be more important? The healthy meal ideas on page 208 should enable you to put the theories into practice in a quick, easy and stress-free way. By looking through them you will see that eating healthily doesn't have to involve more effort than eating unhealthily.

As well as improving children's diet, it's also essential to think about ways of increasing their physical activity level. Too much time spent on sedentary pursuits, such as watching television, is as much to blame as junk food for rising levels of childhood obesity. So there are also a few ideas about how you and your little ones can 'get moving' on page 211.

Even if you do everything right, you'll probably still find some problems with your child's eating occasionally. But then you'd worry if he did eat every healthy meal without question, never asked for anything else and had perfect table manners. So as particular problems arise, deal with them by referring back to the relevant chapters (4–8).

When tackling any difficulties, bear in mind your child's developmental stage as well as his individual personality. Particular solutions will work better with some children than others, and as his parent you are most likely to know what will suit your child, although you might sometimes be surprised by which approach turns out to be effective.

There are some tips at the end of this chapter to help you put all this advice into practice. Before you set out on the journey to improve your child's eating habits, it's important to have realistic expectations about what you can achieve. Then, if you think positively and work together as a family, you'll have happy times as you try to achieve your goals, and not get bogged down by stress.

Ten healthy eating activities

1 The Gimme 5 hand

Get your child to draw around her hand then colour in a finger for each portion of fruit or vegetables she eats today. If she has a banana mid-morning she can colour one finger yellow; if she has a tomato with lunch, that's one red finger. The aim is to fill in all five fingers and make a bright, colourful hand.

2 Plan a meal

Allow your child to plan a lunch or evening meal. He can draw around a plate and do pictures of the foods he wants to include, or he could write a menu. Ask him to choose a protein food, a starchy food and some fruit and/or vegetables. Get him to look in the fridge or cupboards to see if you have all the ingredients, and if there are things to buy, he could help you write a shopping list, or you could go to the shops together.

The first time your child does this, he may well choose to eat something like burger and chips. But by choosing oven chips or potato wedges and burgers with fewest additives (or even homemade ones), the meal needn't be a nutritional disaster. By encouraging him to include vegetables you are teaching him how to make the meal more balanced. Remember always to praise him when he does choose a healthy range of foods. If he rejects the idea of including vegetables, perhaps he could choose some fruit for pudding.

When you sit down to eat, make a point of saying to him

that you are having his dinner, and it should give him a sense of achievement. You could even put up the picture or menu he made.

Make this activity a regular event, perhaps once a week or once a month – depending on how much time you have to do this – but get your child to choose a different meal each time.

3 Going shopping

When you're in the shop ask your child to choose a new fruit or vegetable for all of you to try. Before you go out you could ask her to think about what colour fruit she might like to look for. Make sure you do allow her to choose, even if it's a vegetable you don't know how to cook, and if it is, explain this to her but say that you're willing to give it a go.

If you have an older child, perhaps she could think about how she might choose something to improve her diet. For example, if she usually eats a high-sugar breakfast cereal, get her to look for a lower-sugar one that she could try or mix with the usual variety. Let her read the nutrition information panels to compare the amount of sugar per 100g of each. If she's keen, she could look at fibre too.

4 The label game

This activity is for children who are old enough to read and recognize numbers easily. Get five to 10 foods out of the cupboard – such as cereal, biscuits, baked beans, bread, juice, and so on – then ask your child to put them in order, from the saltiest one down, without looking at the labels. Next, read the labels to see how much salt each one really has per 100g, then reorganize the products.

You could do the same for sugar, fat or fibre, and talk about what each of these do for the body. Explain to your child that he also needs to think about how much of each food he eats; for example, jam has lots of sugar, but he might eat much less of it than, say, frosted cornflakes.

5 Fun with food

Food, particularly healthy food, shouldn't be viewed negatively, so encourage children to have fun with it. They could make a face out of fruit: use slices of kiwi, grapes and satsuma segments to form the eyes, nose, mouth, and hair. Or they could make a house or boat picture, before eating up their artwork. Get them to design a big picture on a serving plate for everyone to enjoy, or an individual one for each member of the family.

6 Pack a picnic

Most children find picnics fun. Get them involved in choosing what to take and in packing it up and they will feel a sense of responsibility. (When the tension of the dinner table is removed in this way, they might be more willing to try new foods.)

7 Food pictures

Choose a nutrient and ask your child to draw foods that

contain it. She could also write down or draw a picture of what the nutrient does: for instance, protein giving her strong muscles or calcium helping her teeth and bones to grow. Of course, children usually enjoy the fibre picture most…

8 Blind tasting

Play a game by putting a blindfold over your child's eyes and giving him a number of foods to taste and identify. Don't offer him foods you know he hates – or he simply won't play. When he's blindfolded, encourage him really to taste the different foods and talk about the flavour and texture. It will help him to think about the more subtle flavours of fresh foods, compared to the over-sweet or salty taste of many processed products.

9 Back to nature

If you have a garden, try growing a few vegetables such as tomatoes, salad leaves or strawberries in a pot. Even if you have only a windowsill you could have a go at growing some cress or planting some herbs or peppers. Alternatively, visit a 'pick-your-own' farm for fruit and vegetables. When children have grown or picked their own produce, you'll find that most will be only too keen to eat it.

10 Cooking together

Cooking with children is absolutely essential for their future well-being; a lack of basic cooking skills is an enormous barrier to healthy eating. It's good to get children started as young as possible, even if they're capable only of making a sandwich.

Ten reasons to cook with your children

1 It's fun.

2 You can easily produce a meal that doesn't contain any added salt, artificial colourings, preservatives, flavourings, or hydrogenated fat, and so on.

3 Children are more likely to try a food if they've been involved in its preparation.

4 It's a cheap form of entertainment.

5 Allergies and other dietary needs can be catered for easily: for instance, by leaving out nuts from a recipe.

6 Cooking builds confidence and a sense of achievement.

7 It provides one-to-one time for chatting. Toddlers are usually keen to talk anyway, but older children (particularly boys) may be reluctant just to sit down for a chat.

8 Using recipes helps with maths, co-ordination, reading and following instructions.

9 By learning a few basic skills children will never have to rely on unhealthy processed foods and take-aways.

10. Before you know it, they'll be making the dinner while you relax with a glass of wine. (Well, you can always dream...)

Ten tips for successful cooking with children

1 Don't expect the end product to look like something Nigella created.

2 Minimize mess with aprons and even cover the floor and the chair – if your child needs one to stand on.

3 Keep safe: remember that small children shouldn't touch sharp knives or cookers.

4 Wash hands and think about hygiene.

5 Keep it simple: don't choose complicated recipes, and make sure you read through each step before starting.

6 If your child gets bored, don't insist she sees it through to the end.

7 Don't just cook cakes – try proper meals such as toppings for pizza bases and making a fruit salad.

8 Talk about different foods, but keep it fun.

9 Let your child get stuck in. He won't do it as well as you, but if he doesn't have a go he'll get bored and won't learn anything.

10 Give lots of praise and encouragement.

Easy family meals

Creating a healthy family meal doesn't have to involve fancy recipes and hours in the kitchen: it's great to try new meals, but you also need a few old favourites which are easy to make and that you know the children will eat. If there are some not-so-healthy meals that your children really enjoy, think about ways you can make them more balanced, such as cooking with less butter, oil, cheese, cream or salt, or by adding extra vegetables.

Ten healthy meal ideas

1   Shepherd's pie with plenty of vegetables, such as carrots and courgettes, in the mince and perhaps with some swede mashed into the potato topping.

2   Stir-fried chicken and vegetables (such as mange-tout, broccoli, spring onions, carrots) and rice.

3   Pasta with a tomato and tuna sauce, made with onions, mushrooms and other vegetables if possible, such as carrots, courgettes or red peppers.

4   Fish fingers, oven chips (buy ones made from just potatoes and oil), peas and carrots.

5   Roast chicken, lamb or other meat with potatoes, broccoli and carrots.

6   Pizza. Homemade or shop-bought bases are good: add toppings (such as mushrooms, peppers, peas or pineapple) and serve with salad or coleslaw on the side.

7   Kedgeree made with rice, salmon, hard-boiled eggs and frozen peas and sweetcorn.

8   Burger (choose ones made from at least 90 per cent beef), ideally in a granary roll, with a few slices of tomato, oven chips and baby corncobs.

9   Cous cous with a mild vegetable and chickpea curry.

10 Vegetable lasagne with plenty of vegetables and not too much cheese.

When you have time to cook, double up the ingredients and make extra batches of pasta sauce or shepherd's pie to put in the freezer as a standby for more hectic days. If you don't have time to cook from scratch and there are no portions left in the freezer, children can still have a reasonably balanced meal with one of the super-quick recipes below. Again, try to make them as healthy as possible by using wholemeal bread, and only a scraping of margarine.

Five super-quick lunches or teas

1   Baked beans on toast, followed by satsumas.

2   Jacket potato with tuna and salad.

3   Cheese and tomato toasted sandwich.

4   Houmous and tzatziki with bits for dipping, such as breadsticks, slices of pitta bread, carrot, cucumber, red pepper or raw mushroom slices.

5   Boiled egg, toast and cherry tomatoes.

Everyday puddings

Most children enjoy something sweet at the end of a meal and it's great if you can make an apple crumble or carrot cake occasionally. For everyday puddings many parents often resort to a 'children's' mousse or jelly, which provides sugar but little else. If offers of fruit or yoghurt are met with a collective moan, try one of the ideas below – they're variations on a theme, but children will find them a lot more appealing.

1   Frozen berries (thawed), topped with natural yoghurt and a sprinkling of muscovado sugar.

2   Mini pots of fruit purée.

3   Kebabs made with fruit, such as strawberries, red grapes, white grapes, sliced banana, tinned pineapple cubes or apricot halves, and marshmallows.

4   Banana lassi made by blending a banana with natural yoghurt and milk.

5   Malt loaf or a jaffa cake with some fresh, tinned or dried fruit on the side, such as raisins, apricots or figs.

Get moving!

Many children spend too much time indoors watching the television or doing other sedentary activities and not enough being physically active. This means they may not use up all the calories they consume and thus they become overweight. However, the benefits of exercise are not limited just to weight control: increasing physical activity also enhances a child's mood and self-esteem (thereby reducing the risk of depression) and it improves sleep quality.

According to NICE (see Resources at the end of the book), children should participate in one hour of moderate activity daily. As well as getting involved in regular activities such as dance, swimming and sports, screen time should be limited and they should be given the opportunity to do something active every day. Physical activity and playing outside should be a part of normal family life. It doesn't matter if your little one isn't the most coordinated child in the world or isn't really interested in sport – you're not trying to set him up to be a top athlete, just fit enough to enjoy a healthy life.

So, in order to get your children moving, try these ideas:

⦾ Limit screen time to an absolute maximum of two hours a day. (That's TV, computer and time spent on electronic games all added together.)

⦾ Go on family outings to the local pool, walk in the woods or ride bikes together.

⦾ Play together outside: for example, fly a kite, or have a game of hide and seek, football, rounders or frisbee.

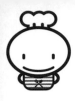

○ If you're going out to eat or visiting the cinema, think about how you can incorporate some physical activity into the outing. Could you visit the park after your meal or walk to the cinema?

○ Show kids how to play hopscotch, tag, stuck in the mud, skipping games or other outdoor activities you enjoyed as a child.

○ Walk more or encourage them to ride their bike or scooter to get around. If you can't walk all the way to school or the shops, try to walk part of the distance.

○ Get your children to join a club or start lessons in some sort of sporting activity, such as swimming, football, martial arts, gymnastics or dancing.

○ Encourage them to beat their personal best, such as in the time it takes to walk around the block or cycle once around the park.

○ Have a disco in the lounge, play musical bumps or get a dance mat.

○ Lead by example.

Tips for moving forward

So you've got this far in the book and you've highlighted your child's problem area. Now it's time to address it and decide how to move forward from it. Sit down and make some plans about how to tackle your child's food issues. But, again, don't try to change too much too quickly.

Set some goals

You might think your child's diet needs a complete overhaul, but even if it does, you need to start by deciding which particular areas to tackle. If you identify specific problems, such as not staying at the table or not eating enough fruit, it becomes easier to find solutions. If you have an impossibly long list, prioritize a simple issue and tackle it first.

Be clear about what you want to achieve and set a specific goal – such as getting your child to eat two portions of fruit a day. If the problem is a particularly difficult one – say, your child refuses to go anywhere near vegetables – you might need a series of goals rather than just the one (see page 102). The first might be simply that your child accepts having a slice of carrot on his plate even though he doesn't taste it. (Look back at the action plan for your particular problem, or at the five dos and don'ts in Chapter 2 for more help.)

Once you have worked out a goal, decide what you're going to do to achieve it and set a specific time frame. For example, for the next month you could help your child do a 'Gimme 5 hand' (see page 202) once a week, offer dried fruit or bananas at breakfast and, if he hasn't eaten two pieces of fruit by tea time, make a fruit pudding. Give yourself a reasonable amount of time for these tactics to work, as it will take a while for everyone to get used to something new.

You may think you are too busy to cook with your child or do some other activity, but if you're serious about getting him to eat well, then you really need to be proactive. Just think about how much effort you spend worrying or nagging about fruit or vegetables and how much better it would be to take a positive approach. We often spend more time thinking about something than actually doing it; it will be more helpful to you if you write down your goals and your plans for achieving them, rather than just thinking about them. When written down in black and white, these targets suddenly become a reality, and even achievable.

Some problems, such as a baby who won't eat lumps, need to be dealt with by you alone, or with your partner if you have one. However, other issues are best tackled with your child. This is particularly true if he is older and has a weight problem, or if he doesn't like milk or vegetables, or some other food.

Realistic expectations

When you are setting a goal you need to think about your other priorities and demands on your time and what you can achieve

It's a good idea to look back regularly at your goals and reassess how your family is doing. If you didn't achieve a previous target, think about whether you aimed too high, or if obstacles got in the way. If this was the case, consider how you might overcome these next time and set new, more realistic, goals. When you do achieve a goal you will feel more positive about everything and it will spur you on to do more.

within these constraints. If you have unrealistically high expectations that you cannot meet, it will most likely leave you with a sense of failure which might make you feel like giving up.

You might decide that you'd like to eat with your children every day, but if they have after-school activities and your partner doesn't get in from work until 7pm, it's not going to happen. However, perhaps you could have breakfast together every day, or lunch and evening meals at the weekend. Or your child might be able to eat a little later, if not every day then perhaps on Friday or Saturday. (Most small children can wait until 6pm or a little later for their dinner, but the benefits of family meals should also be weighed up against the need for children to eat before they're too tired and cranky to enjoy it.) Alternatively, one parent could eat alone one day during the week while the other eats earlier with the children.

If your expectations are too high about the way your child should be eating, you might create some eating problems. While it's not good to eat a bar of chocolate every day, it's okay sometimes. It's not necessarily better, or more virtuous, never to eat chocolate – and this kind of perfectionism can contribute to the development of an eating disorder. If your child is becoming over-concerned with healthy eating or dissatisfied with her looks, pull back a bit. It may be that you are slightly overdoing things. If this is the case you need to make sure you are presenting your child with a balanced approach to food and that you are focusing on her other good qualities, not just her diet or appearance.

Having realistic expectations also means acknowledging that there will be setbacks due to illness, a new baby, problems at school or unexpected late nights at work. You need to accept that these obstacles will get in the way and cope with them as best you can. Setbacks don't mean you need to abandon your plans, just re-work them.

Think positive

Take a positive approach to improving your child's diet and it will seem less daunting. Don't think about 'problems' (which have negative connotations); instead think about 'challenges' that you can rise to and overcome.

If you have a 'can do' attitude, it will not only make you feel better but your enthusiasm will rub off on your children. In the same way, present any changes to them as a pleasure, rather than a chore. Avoid saying you 'should' or 'have to' do something, like more exercise, as it takes all of the joy out of it. Instead say, 'It would be fun' or, 'It would make us feel nice and fit' if we did so and so, such as walked to school more often. Giving your child a small non-food reward (see page 38) might work as an incentive, but be careful how you approach rewards: if your child sees it as a bribe to get him to do something, it might not work so well.

Keep celebrating every success, however small, and it will help you to feel more positive and in control. So, if you manage to achieve your goal of eating with your children two evenings a week, give yourself a pat on the back. If you have a shared

As part of your positive approach, try to withhold criticism and instead look for things to praise your child for. Children really respond well to this approach. So don't say, 'Why aren't you eating the rest of your carrots?' but 'Well done for eating some carrots. I wonder if you'll be able to see better in the dark tonight?'

goal, like walking to school, then you will find that you get a feeling of team achievement whenever you succeed.

Work together and listen

Parents tend to think that they know best and that they have all the answers, but this isn't always the case. In fact, it can be counter-productive to impose strict eating rules on your child. If she is old enough to try to work out a solution to an issue, it's important she gets involved, and if you think of a plan together, she will get a sense of ownership and it will be more likely to succeed.

When you are talking to your child about a problem, try to refrain from taking over the conversation and instead make sure you actively listen to your child's ideas and any objections she may have to your suggestions. Showing you respect her views and think she is capable of intelligent problem-solving will also encourage a sense of responsibility and self-worth in her. This is particularly important if you are tackling a weight problem, as overweight children often suffer from low self-esteem and feel they are unable to control what they do.

Try to help your child to set short-term goals, too, such as eating a banana on the way to school for a week if she refuses breakfast, or walking to school on Tuesday and Thursday. Again, write these down and they will become more real. If you think your little one is setting herself an unrealistic goal, such as cutting down from seven packets of crisps a week to zero, then guide her towards something achievable, like having three packets. If she insists on doing it her way, show your support by going along with the plan, and if she doesn't manage it, don't say, 'I told you so,' but help her to look at the obstacles she experienced and to set a new, more realistic goal.

Similarly, encourage your child to set positive goals, such as eating two pieces of fruit a day or drinking three glasses of water, rather than negatively writing a long list of things not to eat. For some children, self-monitoring is also useful. For example, your child could make a chart and add a sticker for each piece of fruit or glass of water she consumes. Then, when your child achieves her goal it will increase her self-esteem and commitment, and it will also help her grow in confidence and know she can achieve more.

Be consistent

It's important that your approach to feeding your child is balanced and consistent. Once you have decided on particular rules you need to stick to them: it's no good telling your child he must stay at the table for at least 15 minutes while everyone else eats, then letting him get down after five because you can't stand the moaning. It's also important that both parents present a united front – even if you have quite different ideas about how things should be approached. If mum says no eating for an hour before tea, then dad comes home with chocolate, it will inevitably lead to problems.

So if your household includes two parents, you need to decide together what parameters or rules you think are appropriate and feel that you can live with. Then you must agree on a compromise (if necessary) so that you can present a united front. For example, at mealtimes can your child have toys or TV? Must he stay at the table for a set time? Will you insist he tries all foods? What if he doesn't like the food that has been served – will you allow alternatives? If you're unhappy with the amount of sweets, crisps, biscuits or other similar foods that your child eats, you can also think about how often you will allow each of these. It might be that different rules apply in different situations or at the weekend, but considering these issues in advance and deciding how you'll deal with them should reduce arguments and stress.

Ideally, everyone who cares for your child should know about and follow your approach. However, if grandparents insist on indulging their grandchild with treats and they don't actually spend that much time with him it's not worth arguing over. Most children can accept that what goes at Granny's or at a friend's doesn't necessarily apply at home.

A final word

Improving mealtimes can change the whole dynamics of family life, whereby eating can become an enjoyable and social activity that fosters a sense of belonging in your child. So next time you are feeling stressed at teatime, ask yourself whether you can do anything to resolve the situation, or to stop it happening again. If there's nothing you can do, just accept it; but if there is (and there usually is), take action. Remember, being proactive is the antidote to stress.

Don't forget

O Getting your child to eat healthily and happily is an ongoing process; it won't be achieved overnight and new issues
and problems will probably arise.

O If you get your child involved in fun, healthy eating activities, it will help her to understand more about healthy eating,
to be able to make good food choices and to form a healthy
relationship with food.

O Healthy eating needn't be time-consuming and can be
achieved however busy you are – it can even just be about
making small changes to favourite dishes to create more nutritionally balanced meals.

O Children should do one hour of moderate activity every
day. As well as swimming, dancing or taking part in sport,
they need to get more active in everyday life.

O Rise to the 'challenge' that your child's eating habits
present by taking a positive approach and setting realistic
goals.

O Getting older children involved in tackling problems will
increase the chances of success.

O If you take positive action to address problems, you will
automatically feel less stressed.

Resources

Allergies
www.allergyuk.org and Allergy UK Helpline 01322 619898
Advice about dealing with allergies, food intolerance and chemical sensitivity.

Eating disorders
www.b-eat.co.uk and Beat Helpline 0845 634 1414
Information and help from what was formerly known as the Eating Disorders Association.

Nutrition information and advice about feeding
www.babycentre.co.uk
Sensible advice covering pregnancy, babies and toddlers up to 3 years old.

www.bbc.co.uk/parenting and www.bbc.co.uk/health
Expert advice and comments from parents on a variety of topics.

www.foodafactoflife.org.uk
Information for primary school teachers from the British Nutrition Foundation. Also contains great interactive activities for children, such as one for planning a healthy lunchbox.

www.nhsdirect.nhs.uk and helpline 0845 4647
Clear advice and answers to common questions on the website and access to medically trained advisers through a 24-hour hotline.

www.nutrition.org.uk and telephone 020 7404 6504
General advice from the British Nutrition Foundation.

www.foodcom.org.uk
Interesting articles from the Food Commission, which campaigns for safer, healthier food in the UK.

www.fooddudes.co.uk
Information about a programme developed by psychologists at the University of Wales Bangor to get children eating more fruit and vegetables.

www.eatwell.gov.uk
Practical nutrition advice from the Food Standards Agency covering babies and children and including a very helpful ask-the-expert section.

www.mumsnet.com/talk
Help with various aspects of diet, including allergies, and a discussion board for exchanging information with other parents.

Weight problems
www.healthforallchildren.co.uk
Click on child obesity for an online BMI calculator and for percentile charts.

www.nationalobesityforum.org.uk
Information about the prevention and treatment of obesity – including a section specifically about children.

www.nice.org.uk and telephone 020 7067 5800
Guidance on many health issues, including obesity, from the National Institute for Health and Clinical Excellence (NICE).

Vegetarian diets
www.vegansociety.com and telephone 01424 427 393
Health information, recipes and tips for vegans.

www.vegsoc.org and telephone 0161 925 2000
Practical advice about different aspects of vegetarian diets, including diets for babies and children.